Psychiatry, human rights and the law

Psychiatry, human rights and the law

EDITED BY

MARTIN ROTH
*Professor of Psychiatry, University of Cambridge Clinical School
and Fellow of Trinity College, Cambridge*

AND

ROBERT BLUGLASS
Professor of Forensic Psychiatry, University of Birmingham

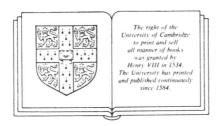

The right of the
University of Cambridge
to print and sell
all manner of books
was granted by
Henry VIII in 1534.
The University has printed
and published continuously
since 1584.

CAMBRIDGE UNIVERSITY PRESS

Cambridge

London New York New Rochelle

Melbourne Sydney

CAMBRIDGE UNIVERSITY PRESS
Cambridge, New York, Melbourne, Madrid, Cape Town, Singapore, São Paulo, Delhi

Cambridge University Press
The Edinburgh Building, Cambridge CB2 8RU, UK

Published in the United States of America by Cambridge University Press, New York

www.cambridge.org
Information on this title: www.cambridge.org/9780521112789

First published 1985
This digitally printed version 2009

A catalogue record for this publication is available from the British Library

Library of Congress Catalogue Card Number: 84-21393

ISBN 978-0-521-26194-4 hardback
ISBN 978-0-521-11278-9 paperback

Contents

Editors' preface

The past twenty-five years have seen rapid change in the manner in which the needs of those suffering from mental illness have been met, in the laws relating to their admission to psychiatric hospitals, and in the treatments administered.

The mid 1950s had been a period of high optimism generated by the introduction of effective new drugs for the treatment of the most serious forms of mental disorder, both in their acute phases and as part of prophylactic management aimed at reducing the chances of relapse. An atmosphere of positive endeavour and high aspiration permeated a large number of mental hospitals and led to the introduction of active programmes of social rehabilitation and resettlement for patients who had, in the past, been all too liable to become residents of such hospitals for years or for life. There was a burgeoning of scientific investigation into the causes and treatment of mental disorder. A group of British mental hospitals had played a pioneering role in these developments and the programmes of management, organization and rehabilitation they employed were emulated in many parts of the world. This movement found expression in the Mental Health Act of 1959 which implemented the main recommendations of the Percy Commission. For ten to fifteen years the Act was regarded as the most humane and imaginative piece of legislation enacted this century in relation to the mentally ill anywhere in the world.

But in the 1970s the Act came under increasing attack as leaving too much scope for medical paternalism. The right given to doctors to administer involuntary treatment to patients whose judgment regarding their best interests may have been impaired or undermined by illness came under particular attack as an infringement of fundamental human rights. The pendulum has swung back, in many countries, to increased legal surveillance and control of the procedures for the compulsory admission of patients to psychiatric hospitals. The right of detained patients to refuse treatment has been incorporated in the legislation enacted in the past decade in several countries, most notably in the United States. It was in this atmosphere of rapid change and intense controversy that ideas incorporated in the Mental Health Act of 1983 germinated and developed.

The Cambridge Conference of which this book is the proceedings, brought together psychiatrists, lawyers, judges, criminologists, social scientists and health administrators; it was held at Trinity College between 1 and 4 September 1983, less than a month before the new Act came into operation on 30 September 1983. It was hoped that the pooling of ideas and the sharing of experiences by scholars and practitioners from six different countries might prove of value and that their contributions in formal papers and discussion be worthy of a wider audience. These hopes have been justified. Some limitations of scope were inevitable, but, in the event, the participants learnt from each other's experiences and ideas and managed to cover a great deal of ground. A few of the themes will be briefly mentioned here by way of introduction.

In the United States 'dangerousness' has become a leading criterion for the admission of mentally ill persons to hospital, displacing from this role the person's need for protection, care and treatment aimed at the restoration of mental well-being. However, used as the only legal and moral justification for involuntary admission it has proved controversial, contentious and an unwieldy instrument in practice. The risk of suicide or danger to others can only be expressed in statistical or actuarial terms aided by clinical judgment; it cannot be 'proved' in a legal sense.

Where courts of law have been given responsibility for arriving at decisions regarding compulsory admission, they have tended to rely on the risk of imminent danger to others as their guideline. However, as they have also proved prone to judge the prediction of risk as wanting in precision for legal purposes, the selection of cases for commitment has become an arbitrary process and the law has seemed, in such settings, to have entered an era of confusion. There is a mounting volume of protest against the growing number of violent attacks by the mentally ill and personality-disordered discharged from hospital into some of the large cities of the world.

The right of the mentally ill to punishment for any offences committed, rather than confinement in a psychiatric hospital on an indeterminate basis, has in recent years been increasingly asserted as an inalienable human right. It is generally accepted that patients should not be sequestered for long periods following trivial offences such as simple exhibitionism or obscene telephone calls merely because a psychiatric diagnosis has at one time been attached to them. Yet, when an individual has committed repeated arson or an act of poisoning or a number of sexual murders, some estimate of the risk for society and an objective, fair and compassionate judgment of what action might be taken to minimize it, is inescapable. Neither short nor long sentences nor the substitution of 'punishment' for 'treatment' will dispose of the problem. In its essence, it is far older than the disciplines of psychiatry or the law.

The rift between psychiatry and the law has been reflected in dramatic manner in the United Kingdom in the trials and in the judgments pronounced in the cases of Sutcliffe (the 'Yorkshire Ripper') and Nielsen, and in the trial of President Reagan's would-be assassin, Hinckley, in the United States. These are merely well-publicized examples drawn from a multitude of others in which a growing divergence between the philosophies and the practices of the two intellectual diciplines and social institutions has become manifest in recent years. Although the insanity defence has been accepted in its essentials since the beginnings of recorded history, demands for its abolition or redefinition have been increasingly voiced and implemented in the last few decades. Lord Devlin has complained that 'everywhere the concept of illness expands continually at the expense of the concept of moral responsibility'. There are, indeed, real problems inherent in the insanity defence and the difficult concept of diminished responsibility. But examination of the historical record makes it plain that these problems are also ancient and not the creation of psychiatrists, lawyers or any particular form of social organization.

Twenty-five years ago, the evils of institutionalization provided the main target for the critics of psychiatry. This has changed to the hardships imposed by 'de-institutionalization' or 'de-carceration'. In the United Kingdom, the number of psychiatric beds has been halved in the past quarter of a century. But many patients with chronic illness have been discharged into communities who care little, or not at all. Some return home to inflict hardships on relatives, whilst others can be seen wandering homeless and aimless in city streets. When refused admission to hospital after committing minor offences, they are sentenced to terms of imprisonment contributing substantially to the serious overcrowding of the prisons and the depersonalization of those condemned to inhabit them.

The Cambridge Conference considered possible approaches towards resolving the main dilemmas that face psychiatry, society and the law in healing the rifts that have arisen between the professions concerned with the care of the mentally ill. It sought, also, to learn from past errors and consider means for the promotion of more humane, successful and socially efficient mental health and prison services. The Conference was made possible by the generosity of the late Baron ver Heyden de Lancey, who endowed a Fund for the encouragement of medico-legal studies at Trinity College, Cambridge. He took great interest in the Conference, but was unable to attend owing to failing health. It is sad that his death in the past year should have denied him the satisfaction of seeing the consummation of its work in the publication of this volume.

August 1984   M.R.
                                                        R.B.

Contributors

Robert Bluglass, Professor of Forensic Psychiatry, Midland Centre for
  Forensic Psychiatry, All Saints Hospital, Birmingham B18 5SD, UK
Robert J. Campbell, Director, Gracie Square Hospital, Gracie Square,
  Manhattan, New York, USA
Jean Floud, Former Principal, Newnham College, Cambridge CB3 9DF, UK
Larry Gostin, National Association for Mental Health, 22 Harley Street,
  London W1N 2ED, UK
John Gunn, Professor of Forensic Psychiatry, Institute of Psychiatry,
  De Crespigny Park, Denmark Hill, London SE5 8AF, UK
John R. Hamilton, Medical Director, Broadmoor Hospital, Crowthorne,
  Berkshire RG11 7EG, UK
H. Helmchen, Head, Psychiatrische Klinik und Poliklinik der Freien
  Universität Berlin, Eschenallee 3, D-1000 Berlin 19, Federal Republic of
  Germany
Villars Lunn, Professor of Psychiatry, Institute of Psychiatry, The Royal
  State Hospital, Copenhagen, Denmark
William H. Reid, Associate Professor of Psychiatry and Director of Education
  and Training, Nebraska Psychiatric Institute, University of Nebraska
  Medical Centre, 602 South 45th Street, Omaha, Nebraska 68106, USA
Martin Roth, Professor of Psychiatry, University of Cambridge Clinical
  School, Level 4, Addenbrooke's Hospital, Hills Road, Cambridge CB2
  2QQ
P. Sarteschi, Professor of Psychiatry, Institute of Clinical Psychiatry,
  University of Pisa, Via Roma 67, Pisa, Italy
Margaret A. Somerville, Professor, Faculty of Law and Faculty of Medicine,
  McGill University, 3644 Peel Street, Montreal, PQ, Canada H3A 1W9
Alan A. Stone, Professor of Law and Psychiatry, Faculty of Law and Faculty
  of Medicine, Harvard University, Cambridge, Mass. 02138, USA
Nigel Walker, Wolfson Professor of Criminology, Institute of Criminology,
  West Road, Cambridge, UK
Sir John Wood, Professor of Law, Faculty of Law, University of Sheffield,
  Crookesmoor Building, Sheffield S10 2TN, UK

The historical background: the past 25 years since the Mental Health Act of 1959

MARTIN ROTH

The late 1950s was a time of rapid progress in the treatment of psychiatric disorder, liberal legislation in mental health and expansion of research into the causes of mental illness along a broad front. Drugs that were effective in treating depressive illness had been recently discovered and their applications in clinical practice spread with an unprecedented rapidity. The Percy Commission was coming to the end of its deliberations, and the English Mental Health Act of 1959 which followed has been widely described as this century's most humane piece of legislation in relation to the mentally ill to be placed on the statute books anywhere. The prospects for better mutual understanding between the law and psychiatry were full of high promise.

The changes that followed the creation of more stimulating and active regimes in psychiatric wards and the successes of new treatments for depression, schizophrenia and other disorders generated a fresh upsurge of scientific investigation into the biological and social origins of mental illness. The steep decline in the number of beds in English mental hospitals which began in 1954 intensified the atmosphere of optimism. There had been 344 beds per 100000 population at the end of 1954. This was halved to 171 per 100000 by 1978. The total number of mental hospital beds in England was reduced from 160000 to 80000 in the same period. The reduction was due in part to the discharge of patients who had been resident in mental hospitals for many years, but to a greater extent to a decrease in the average length of stay of patients. This was the beginning of the era of the revolving door. But the Department of Health in this country was already looking with confidence to the closure of the large mental hospitals and the creation of small psychiatric units in district general hospitals where the treatment of patients with acute mental illness was mainly to be undertaken in future. The tasks of the mental health services were to be discharged in the community, where those with chronic illnesses were to be protected from the dangers of institutionalization. A number of these developments had been inspired by the philosophy underlying the Mental Health Act of 1959. Most patients with psychiatric disorder were in future to be admitted without compulsion or formality.

The patients were to enjoy the same privileges and consideration as did those with physical illness, able to enter or leave hospital by their own free choice and to accept or refuse treatment offered to them. In that limited group of patients whose illness rendered them incapable of judging the risks they faced or the treatments they needed, treatment could be arranged on a compulsory basis, but without the intervention of magistrates or courts of law. Authority for the admission of such patients, who made up 10.1% of the total in 1979 (DHSS Consultative Document), was vested entirely in medical hands and it remains in medical hands in the Mental Health Act of 1983 which is described in detail by Professor Bluglass.

Antipsychiatrists and their allies

The clear vision of the future of mental health services and the high optimism and confidence that characterize the Percy Report were even then being eroded by attacks from several directions. All procedures for the care, admission and treatment of patients with mental disorders were soon to be assailed as infringements of basic human rights.

The different lines of attack were inter-related. The antipsychiatry of Szasz, Laing, Esterson and Foucault alleges that mental illnesses are not illnesses but socially deviant behaviours. In Foucault's version, the function of psychiatry is to exercise control over deviants whose 'radical voices' threaten the existing social order. Psychiatry is an instrument of coercion employed by the ruling classes against those who dissent from or revolt against society's established rules and conventions. As an ideology, it obscures and mystifies the nature of power struggles within society which are resolved by one-sided, arbitrary and repressive means. A similar critique has been advanced along other fronts. In the 1980 Reith Lectures the lawyer Ian Kennedy (1981) declared that the expertise of psychiatrists consists of 'the exercise of moral, social and political judgments concerning the worth of someone's thinking'. What passes as mental illness is for the most part no more than politically subversive ideas, protests against racial injustice or deviant sexual behaviour. It is the metaphor of illness that enables the thought-policemen to deprive the individual of liberty without due process of law or adequate right of appeal. In the Utopian writings of Ivan Illich the attack is extended to the entire practice of medicine. The quest for health and health services is described as a monolithic world religion, the subversion of which would advance the cause of human well-being.

Fringe medicine and the claims of homeopaths, chiropractors, osteopaths and practitioners of mystical cults who offer to relieve pain and disease and promote positive health are currently much debated in the news media and the glossy magazines. 'Alternative' medicine is fashionable and is patronized by the highest in this and other lands, and has recently been given the solemn imprimatur of a first leader in *The Times* and the blessing of a member of the Royal Family.

A succession of scandals in England and elsewhere which have originated from neglect, inhumane treatment or abuse of psychiatric patients in mental hospitals have been used to buttress the case of the antipsychiatric and human rights lobbies. Psychiatrists are described in this literature as favouring compulsion; but the historical record shows that they have often been in the vanguard of liberal reform in mental health legislation for almost two centuries.

Mental health issues in the political arena

It is not clear why the subject of mental health should in recent times have become politicized in theory and practice through neo-Marxist analysis and the advocacy of the civil rights lobby. The view that the emergence of psychiatry as a medical discipline was closely related to the evolution of capitalist society proves to bear little relationship to fact. Recent research has shown that since the beginnings of recorded history societies have recognised certain disordered states of mind as mental illness and given the profession of medicine responsibility for treating them.

Mental illness, was for example, a well-recognized condition in the Near East in 1000 BC. In the Old Testament David, fearing for his life when captured by the Philistines wearing the sword of Goliath, feigns lunacy, banging on doors and letting spittle run down his beard. His strategy was wholly successful, for the King of the Philistines diagnosed insanity and refrained from causing harm to a madman even though an enemy. During the Middle Ages, contrary to the standard histories of the period, lay and clerical physicians continued by practice and teaching to uphold an ancient humane tradition of medical care of the mentally ill. This flourished alongside the cruel persecutions of the insane that stemmed from beliefs in demonology and witchcraft about which so much has been written. Medical scholarship and healing were kept alive within the monasteries throughout the Dark Ages, extending outwards from the cathedral schools after the eleventh and twelfth centuries (Kroll, 1973). The medical take-over of the asylum and the invention of mental illness at the end of the seventeenth century in the interest of bourgeoning capitalism – the teaching of Foucault and Scull – can hardly be reconciled with such findings.

The oscillation between hospital and community care

The last 140 years have seen alternation between care of the mentally ill in hospital and care in the community. In the last century pychiatric patients in the care of the inhumane local authorities were transferred with great ceremony to the new mental hospitals which were to cure them with the aid of moral treatment. Charles Dickens, visiting the United States at the start of this era, was very impressed with a small mental hospital where the superintendent and staff sat down with the patients for meals. The patients ate with knives and forks, enjoyed carriage drives and engaged in productive work in an attempt to rebuild their self-respect. Now, on an equally triumphant note, patients are being transferred in large number from the hospitals which allegedly caused their condition to deteriorate, back into the community. But the community rarely cares, and the facilities provided have proved sadly inadequate. The presence of the whole necessary range of supervised hostels, sheltered housing, adequate medical care, occupation, retraining and rehabilitation within a community service is a very rare exception. In some countries the predicament of families has become desperate. Some of the multitude of patients set adrift in the large cities of the world come into conflict with the law, and when hospitals refuse to admit them they are sent to prison. This is one road leading to the criminalization of the mentally ill.

In the writings of antipsychiatrists these trends are depicted as the evils of 'incarceration' and the even greater iniquities of 'decarceration', that is, the release of patients in large number into unprepared communities. But as Professor Kathleen Jones (1982), has cogently said, ' If it is wrong to get patients out of mental hospital, and wrong to keep them in, what are we to do with them?' The fact is that such obdurate and painful dilemmas are not to be resolved or spirited away with the aid of any known social, medical, political or administrative remedies.

The right to receive and the right to refuse treatment

We are caught in uncertainty between the poles of another antithesis when we turn to rights relative to treatment. The right of patients confined in mental hospitals to receive treatment has been enshrined in a number of important decisions in the United States in particular (*Rouse* v. *Cameron*, 1966; *Wyatt* v. *Stickney*, 1971; *O'Connor* v. *Donaldson*, 1975). The problem of defining what constitutes adequate treatment in different types of disorder is not solved.

The right to treatment can run into head-on collision with the right to refuse treatment, also established in law: if the patient has a legal entitlement to adequate care, has he also the right to receive treatment under compulsion when suffering from depression with grave suicidal risk? The implementation of this right is demanded in some cases by spouses, children and relatives, and by patients between attacks of periodic illness. Manic-depressive patients, whose insight often returns in the course of a remission, may give instructions to their psychiatrists that when they refuse treatment during illness, appropriate action should be taken to protect their lives. There are clear and well-established indices of suicidal danger in patients and when they have not been heeded the responsible psychiatrist is liable to be sued for negligence by relatives seeking redress and compensation.

The problem with principles and doctrines such as the right to refuse treatment is that they advance simplistic solutions to problems of a complex and obdurate nature. To take up just one thread in a whole web of causes and consequences, there are the human rights of dependent wives, children and parents to be considered as well as those of the patient.

But in spite of all these reservations recent developments in attitudes to psychiatric treatment are a forward step. In an increasing number of countries it is being clearly spelt out that treatment should normally proceed only on the basis of the full consent of those competent to give it. In some legislation it is also explicit that, except in emergency, the refusal of those manifestly incompetent to give consent must not be overridden unless an independent assessment confirms that treatment is essential to preserve life or conserve health.

Mental illness and morality

Criticisms have often been voiced in the past 25 years regarding the extent to which the concept of illness has increasingly encroached upon and usurped the territory that was once the exclusive province of morality. Not only conditions crudely subsumed in the past under the heading of 'madness' but all forms of psychiatric disorder were assimilated into 'illness'. And it was implied that only those free from psychiatric taint were regarded by psychiatrists as fully answerable and responsible for their antisocial deeds. Under the Durham laws in the United States some 30 years ago, psychiatric illness was given a very wide definition and advocacy within the adversarial system contributed to widen it even further. It was pleaded in some cases that conditions that go under the name of personality disorder could in themselves give rise to the same global disturbance with distorted perception of the world, derangement of motivation and impaired control over conduct as do psychoses such as schizophrenia. The repute and standing of psychiatry and psychiatric testimony in court inevitably suffered. In Europe a much stricter definition of psychiatric illness survived, as Professor Lunn discusses in his paper. In Denmark's Medico-Legal Council only those offenders diagnosed as psychotic are likely to be judged not punishable and sent to a mental hospital. Different judgments are pronounced in cases of personality disorder and psychopathy.

The inverse care law in psychiatric services

The 'inverse care law' refers to the situation in which the needs of substantial groups of patients with severe forms of psychiatric disorder prove to be inversely proportionate to the location of the facilities required for their treatment or long-term care. It comes into operation by a number of different routes. In the United Kingdom psychiatric hospitals are given the right to refuse admission to patients who are regarded as being unsuited to the facilities available. In consequence a relatively large number of highly disturbed, aggressive and difficult patients have been denied admission to ordinary psychiatric hospitals. Some have had to be accepted in Broadmoor or other maximum security hospitals, which are often inappropriate and which have become appallingly overcrowded. Others end in prison. The Butler Committee recommended that the majority of such cases be accommodated within special secure units to be created within each region. Very few have been established, and a proportion of the patients who should be in such units are adrift in the large cities, asleep under bridges, in doorways or in the corners of railway stations.

In other countries the situation develops by a different route. In the United States dangerousness appears to have become the criterion employed by the courts in deciding whether compulsory admission of mentally disturbed patients is justified. This criterion survives despite the repeated insistence of many legal authorities that the prediction of dangerousness is a highly unreliable exercise. Be this as it may only a small proportion of psychotic patients are dangerous and therefore qualify for admission to hospital. The majority are consequently denied the treatment they often need as a matter of urgency. Those admitted contain a relatively high proportion of patients with serious personality disorder passing through a phase of explosive conduct complicated by alcohol abuse, drug dependence or both. There are no effective treatments available for such patients and hospital can provide only a 'cooling-off' period while their condition reaches a more quiescent stage. The net result is that those cases where management in an ordinary psychiatric hospital is of little avail or can have only a transient effect cause such hospitals to strain at the seams, while many of those in need of a specific treatment that would be likely to help them to remission do not receive care.

Concluding remarks

The number of psychiatric beds has fallen steeply during the past 25 years. Almost half a century ago Lionel Penrose (1939) demonstrated an inverse correlation in the countries of Europe between prison places and psychiatric beds: the smaller the number of psychiatric beds (the only psychiatric facilities available at that time) the larger the number of prison places. A high ratio of the number of patients in mental hospitals as against the number of those confined in prisons has in the past been regarded as one index of progress towards more humane, enlightened and non-primitive attitudes within societies. As far as the mentally ill are concerned the clock has, by this criterion, been put back. For care in the community which was intended to fill the gap created by closure or contraction of the mental hospitals has been found wanting almost everywhere.

A little over 130 years ago, on 25 November 1853, Sir John Bucknill, writing in the first issue of the *Asylum Journal* (later to become the *Journal of Mental Science*), paid tribute to Pinel who had 'vindicated the rights of science against the usurpations of superstition and brutality and rescued the victims of mental disease from the exorcist and the gaoler'. He went on to state that the physician had become the responsible guardian of those with mental disorder and that he must remain so, adding with unshakable confidence and Victorian thunder 'unless by some calamitous reverse the progress of the world and civilisation should be arrested and turn back in the direction of practical barbarism'.

Now, 130 years later, exorcism is still with us, the mentally ill are to be found in large numbers in prisons of every kind, the 'medical model' of mental illness and all models bearing any kinship to it are under attack from many quarters. 'Alternative' forms of medicine thrive and a whole range of new religions have attracted converts and earthly riches through their promises of tranquillity and identity to large numbers of young people who have felt bereft of them. One objective of the conference was

to promote better understanding and to rebuild bridges between disciplines that should be working in cooperation at the interface between the
medical, social and legal aspects of mental disorders.

A further purpose was to extract some of the lessons learned during a
period of 25 years that has seen more rapid and radical changes than any
other quarter-century since the start of the debate between medicine,
society and the law about the problems posed by mental disorder. New
laws are already being administered in a number of countries and it is to be
hoped that they will be able to draw upon the conclusions reached by the
many groups of medical and legal scholars, criminologists, philosophers
and social scientists who have come together as they did in Cambridge in
1983 to pool their knowledge and observations and to distil the experience
of what proves to have been a revolutionary era in the history of the mental
health movement. They have worked in the hope that the insights gained
may be applied with benefit when the winds of change commence to blow
afresh in relation to the organisation of services for the mentally ill, the
legal provisions made by societies for their care and for protection of their
human rights, and the proper roles of medicine and the law within those
areas of psychiatry in which problems of common concern for both
disciplines are frequently posed.

REFERENCES

Bucknill, J. (1853). *The Asylum Journal.*
Jones, K. (1982). Scull's dilemma. *British Journal of Psychiatry*, 141, 221–6.
Kennedy, I. (1981). *The Unmasking of Medicine.* (Based on the Reith
    Lectures, 1980.) London: Allen and Unwin.
Kroll, J. (1973). A reappraisal of psychiatry in the Middle Ages. *Archives of
    General Psychiatry*, 29, 276–83.
O'Connor v. *Donaldson*, 43 USLW 4929 (1975).
Penrose, L.S. (1939). Mental disease and crime: outline of a comparative
    study of European statistics. *British Journal of Medical Psychology*, 18,
    1–15.
Roth, M. and Kroll, J. (1985). *The Reality of Mental Illness.* Cambridge
    University Press (in press).
Rouse v. *Cameron*, 373 F.2d 451 (D.C. Cir. 1966).
Scull, A.T. (1975). From madness to mental illness: medical men as moral
    entrepreneurs. *Archives européennes de Sociologie*, 16, 218–51.
Wyatt v. *Stickney*, 325. F. Supp. 781, 748 (M.D. Ala. 1971).

The social and medical consequences of recent legal reforms of mental health law in the USA: the criminalization of mental disorder

ALAN A. STONE

During the decade of the eighties, two images of mental illness have come to dominate the public imagination and the mass media in the United States. One image is of the violent, paranoid killer. This is the image featured on the evening news. John Hinckley's attack on President Reagan is perhaps the most famous example. It has been shown all over the world and has been replayed scores of times in the United States. Hinckley was under the care of a psychiatrist at the time. This and other similar cases have focussed media attention on the alleged negligence of psychiatrists in allowing these insane killers to go free. John Lennon's killer left a mental hospital in Hawaii, travelled to New York, and gunned down his victim. An acutely psychotic man released from a Massachusetts state hospital travelled to Florida and decapitated an innocent young boy. A man sent home on a visit from a New York state hospital, killed the wife he had been threatening to kill. This image of violent insanity unleashed by incompetent psychiatrists blends into that other familiar image of violent crime: mugging, rape, murder – crime in the streets.

Whatever the explanation for these kinds of violence, whether it is madness or badness, it is clear that the American public now wants more protection. Many Americans feel betrayed by the criminal justice system and in addition there is a growing public feeling that incompetent psychiatrists and radical civil libertarians have together deprived the public of a measure of much-needed protection and unleashed maniacs on society. Is the American public correct? Are they now more at risk? If so, is it because of incompetent psychiatrists and because of civil libertarians who care more about the rights of maniacs than the lives of victims? I shall come back to these questions, but here I want to anticipate. Incompetent psychiatrists are a problem, and some of the lurid examples above are instances of incompetence, but all psychiatrists are incompetent when they are assigned tasks beyond their abilities. And, of course, new procedural safeguards for the mentally ill increase the risks that the dangerous mentally ill will go free. The significance of procedural safeguards is to increase the burden of the state in making its case for confinement.

The other eighties image of mental illness in the United States is typified by the 'bag lady'. The public sees her wandering the streets of all our major cities – distracted, dishevelled, homeless, and acting peculiarly. Decades ago one could safely assume that the majority of derelicts were alcoholics. Now one can assume that 50 to 75% of the homeless are chronic psychiatric patients – the deinstitutionalized.[1] Although some citizens are frightened by the sight of this new class of derelicts, there is also a feeling of shame and outrage when one sees an elderly lady sleeping in the doorway of an office building or rummaging through trash cans. Where is the Government's vaunted safety net of welfare services? Who is getting her social security checks? Where are her food stamps? Why isn't someone taking care of her? Where is her social worker, her psychiatrist, her lawyer?

The first image of madness, the violently insane, points up the failure of public protection, and the second image of madness, the 'bag lady', suggests the failure of public responsibility. Public protection – the police power – and public responsibility – *parens patriae* – are of course the underlying legal justifications for civil commitment, and these two images of the eighties seem therefore to demonstrate the failure of both of those objectives. In fact, these images of madness in the eighties are a reflection of American legal reforms in the seventies. They are a second generation of problems created by attempts to solve a first generation of problems.

But these public images of madness do not tell the whole story of the failures of legal reform in the United States. There is a tragic set of private images known to those who have a child, a spouse, or a parent who is mentally ill. Consider the following case example which is a fair composite of several cases I have dealt with in the past decade.

Mr X is a 23-year-old law student. He has worked hard to get into law school and his family have worked hard to support his education. During the second semester of his first year, his classmates notice that Mr X has begun to act strangely. He arrives early in class, takes the seat closest to the professor and fixes him with an angry and intimidating glare. Over the course of the next few days the student's behavior becomes more objectionable. He interrupts his classes with incoherent tirades. He refuses to leave classes when asked to by his professor. He looks increasingly dishevelled and students avoid sitting next to him because he smells bad. By now 150 of his classmates are convinced that something is terribly wrong with Mr X. Either he is having a 'problem in living' as some have labeled it or he has begun to demonstrate symptoms of a serious mental illness. In the years before the 'criminalization of civil commitment' this young man could have been hospitalized against his 'will' at this point. Now a psychiatrist has no authority to do this because involuntary confinement requires proof beyond a reasonable doubt that the person is mentally ill and dangerous to self or others. Several of his classmates approach Mr X and suggest that he voluntarily seek help of various kinds. He refuses and makes veiled references to a conspiracy in which they are involved. The Assistant Dean calls Mr X to his office and suggests that he not go to class until he can control his tirades. He also urges the student to see a psychiatrist or contact his parents, even offering to call them himself, but Mr X angrily objects that he is an adult and wants nothing to do with psychiatry or his parents. Over the next week the situation deteriorates still further. The student turns up in classes all over the law school – classes in which he is not even enrolled. He takes his special seat, glares at the professors, and interrupts the classes with incoherent tirades. By now it is clear to at least 30 law professors and 1000 law students that something is radically wrong with Mr X.

It is sometimes said, as it was by the Federal courts of the United States, that psychiatric hospitalization is stigmatizing and alleged patients must be and are protected by the Constitution from the power of psychiatrists to impose that stigma.[2] But in this case, at least, the young man was becoming stigmatized as a result of his own symptomatic actions. It is also sometimes said, as it was by these same Federal judges, that it is psychiatric hospitalization, *per se*, that makes it difficult to get a job. But in this case, at least, the young man was probably damaging his future employment opportunities because he was not hospitalized. The Federal judges of Wisconsin who authored the benchmark decision, *Lessard* v. *Schmidt* (1972),[3] criminalizing civil commitment gave as a prime example of career damage and stigma an elected official much in the news at that time. Senator Eagleton had been deprived of his opportunity to stand as a candidate for Vice President in George McGovern's campaign because of the stigma of his psychiatric hospitalization. No doubt in a certain sense the judges are correct, but what would Senator Eagleton's career have been like – what would the stigma have been – if he had not been hospitalized and treated appropriately? Our Federal judges influenced by the ideology of antipsychiatry could not conceive of the need to balance the stigma of untreated illness against the stigma of treated illness.

At any rate, to get back to my example, the law school Dean decided to call Mr X's parents. Although they came at once, much to their surprise there was nothing they could do. Under the law they were powerless. There is no authority under which they could get their son to a psychiatrist or to a hospital, and all their pleas to him were rejected. They went to see the school's psychiatrist who had already been consulted by the Dean. He informed them that under the new state laws on civil commitment there was nothing that he, the psychiatrist, could do unless their son was dangerous to himself or others or was so gravely disabled that he could not take care of his basic needs for food and shelter. When it seemed there was nothing else to be done to help the law student, and after warning the student of the consequences, the law school took official disciplinary action and suspended him. Mr X refused to acknowledge the suspension and continued to attend classes. One week later, this young student, who by now was obviously hallucinating, deluded, and in the throes of a severe psychotic episode, was barred from entering a classroom by the Dean. The student pushed him aside and was then seized by the campus police. He had now met the objective legal standard: he was mentally ill and dangerous to others as manifested by a past act – pushing the Dean.

What I have described to you is not a case that interests our national media. But I believe it should be of interest to those who promulgate mental health laws. It is a case of needless suffering, both for the student and his family. It is an example of what American psychiatrists now confront as they struggle to cope with the second generation of problems created by the law-givers who rejected the 'paternalistic medical model' of psychiatric hospitalization.

But the difficulties of this case are not over. Although the law student now is subject to emergency certification there will be a probable cause hearing with procedural safeguards. In some jurisdictions he cannot be medicated until the hearing and this alleged patient must be assigned a lawyer whose task is to be a zealous advocate for liberty and not someone who decides whether hospitalization is in his client's best interest. The student does not want to be hospitalized and he does not want to be treated. He tells his lawyer these are not his real parents; they are substitutes. He claims it is all a conspiracy. They are reading his mind; references are made to him on television; he is being persecuted. What will his zealous advocate do in the face of all this psychotic ideation? The courts instruct the lawyer to be a zealous advocate for liberty: he must fight the civil commitment, assert the young man's right to refuse treatment! What will the judge do? Will he stick to the letter of the law? It is my claim that if the lawyer is a zealous advocate and if the judge does stick to the letter of the law, there is a good chance this student will be discharged untreated.

The purpose of the new civil commitment laws as applicable in this case, is to confine people who are mentally ill and dangerous. But this student has only pushed the Dean and that only because he barred his way. Like most people who have acute psychotic disorders, he is probably not really a danger to society. Although it is possible to prove beyond a reasonable doubt that he pushed the Dean, it is not possible to prove he is still dangerous. Every empirical study of the prediction of dangerousness demonstrates that psychiatrists, psychologists, and computers cannot accurately identify which psychotic patients are the dangerous persons.[4] A zealous advocate can make a convincing argument that the alleged patient, even if he was slightly dangerous when he pushed the Dean, is certainly no longer really dangerous. He can also advise his client not to talk to the psychiatrists and encourage him to assert his right to remain silent. The courts of some jurisdictions have ruled that the alleged patient like the alleged criminal has Fifth Amendment rights. The lawyer can, as a zealous advocate, preserve his client's liberty and prevent his treatment.

The American system of adversarial justice is based on the premise that there are legal advocates on both sides. We understand the incentives for balanced advocacy when the state has to prosecute criminals, but what is the state's incentive to use scarce prosecutorial resources to press for the confinement and treatment of this law student? Does it really make sense for the public prosecutors to engage in costly litigation in order to confine this young man so that the state can then spend $200 a day to treat him? Remember, American prosecutors are elected officials who now do not have sufficient legal staff and resources to try the vast numbers of criminals who threaten society.

And what of the psychiatrists? The wave of legal reform which we are discussing seems to have been premised on the assumption that psychiatrists were persons of enormous power and determination who had to be restrained by new laws and an active mental health bar. Some legal reformers were misled by radical critics of psychiatry and their dire prophecies about the therapeutic state. But psychiatrists have never had a great interest in civil commitment; it was an unpleasant obligation, not an enjoyable exercise of power. Legal writers have repeatedly noted that psychiatrists, when they are challenged about civil commitment or are told there will be a lengthy hearing on a particular case, will often change their minds and back off. This kind of reaction is often cited as evidence of the arbitrariness and unreliability of psychiatric diagnosis and decision making. This, I think, is an unfortunate misinterpretation. On the one hand I believe it reflects the general psychiatric antipathy to participation in civil commitment. Most psychiatrists, after all, have neither the training nor the temperament to be implacable prosecutors. Nor do most psychiatrists want to spend time in the courtroom matching wits with lawyers. If the state has no great incentive for civil commitment of patients, the vast majority of psychiatrists have no stomach for it. The Orwellian vision of Big Brother and 1984 was a false prophecy. What we have instead in the United States are huge inept public mental health bureaucracies which cannot keep track of their own employees never mind their 'clients'. In the end, the only ones who really care about the law student I have described are his parents.

But there is now built into mental health law in the United States an assumption of a conflict of interests between the family and the alleged patient like Mr X.[5] The zealous legal advocate protects his client from parental attempts to get him treated. The family is condemned to watch their psychotic son get worse and worse without assistance. How long will it be before they give up in helplessness? How long will it be before the legal activists demand that a new class of bureaucrats be funded by the legislature to serve as guardians for such patients to protect them from their relatives' interference? How long will it be before the newspapers are reporting neglect and abuse by these public guardians? This is not an imaginary scenario; it has already happened in the United States.[6]

During the past decade, I have been repeatedly consulted by family members about patients like Mr X. There is little hope one can offer them; their tragic situation is part of the second generation of problems created by legal reform. The fate of most people with serious chronic mental illness is that they end up alone, abandoned by family and by friends. Hollingshead and Redlich[7] demonstrated this circumstance 25 years ago and every experienced clinician can confirm it from his or her practice. Legal reforms will, I am afraid, contribute to this abandonment.

Thus far I have presented three images of madness. The dangerous maniac and the deinstitutionalized derelict are the two media images. The less well publicized problem is the person with an acute psychotic disorder who is suffering, is ruining his own life, and is causing great suffering to his family. I do not mean to exaggerate the numbers in this third category. Eventually, many will seek help voluntarily. But there are some, like the law student Mr X, who will not, as a result of reforms such as those authored by the Federal courts of the United States.

It may be worth taking a closer look at those legal reforms and the first generation of problems they aimed at solving.

During 1960, one out of every 300 Americans was involuntarily confined in a mental institution. Many of those institutions were not only inadequate, they were harmful. Doctor Harry Solomon, President of the American Psychiatric Association, declared in 1958 that the state hospitals were 'bankrupt beyond remedy'. The institutions for the criminally insane were still worse and those who worked at that time, as I did, in institutions for the mentally retarded could say that they were even more awful. Clearly something was terribly wrong with the way American society was dealing with the mentally disabled.

The question was what to do about it. There were two kinds of reform mounted in the sixties. One came from within psychiatry: the philosophy of community mental health, which aimed at dismantling the state hospitals and providing quality care in local treatment facilities. The advent of effective medication, the emerging policy of short-term treatment, revolving door admissions, and partial hospitalization changed a great deal. But the grand strategy was never fully implemented, for reasons I cannot discuss here. However, one result of these psychiatric reforms is crucial to our discussion of civil commitment. In 1958, the average length of hospitalization for patients diagnosed as schizophrenic was 13.1 years.[8] Today the length of hospitalization is measured in days or weeks rather than in years. We send the patients back to the community, but we have only grudgingly admitted that there *is* no community. The greatest iatrogenic problem of the mental health system today is the failure of continuity of care – legal reform has allowed us to rationalize our failures.

The second kind of reform of the mental health system came from the law. It was inspired by three complementary perspectives exemplified by the case I discussed. One perspective was that of the civil libertarians. They argued, in effect, that the mental patient should have the same procedural safeguards as the criminal. The patient became an 'alleged patient' and the psychiatrist was treated as the legal equivalent of a policeman. I have called this 'the criminalization of civil commitment'. That was the approach followed by our Federal courts in the benchmark case of *Lessard* v. *Schmidt*. I shall have more to say about that later.

The second perspective inspiring legal reform emphasized the inadequacies of psychiatric treatment and the terrible conditions in the hospitals. The establishment of this approach as a legal tradition began with the famous Gault decision of the United States Supreme Court dealing with juvenile delinquents.[9] Justice Abe Fortas, reviewing the horrible failure of rehabilitative institutions for juveniles, concluded that Gault and other juveniles should have more due process safeguards. Justice would be done if the state had more legal hurdles to overcome and the juvenile more procedural protection before being confined in these appalling institutions. To a psychiatrist this seems like a strange remedy. It is rather like the health department deciding that rather than close a restaurant that is serving contaminated food until the contamination is removed, it will bar four of the eight entrances. The result in the United States Juvenile System is well known; rehabilitation facilities for juveniles remain a national disgrace. The Supreme Court's additional due process safeguards are met and juveniles are sent to institutions where they become socialized as criminals. If a mental hospital cannot provide adequate treatment, then it makes no sense to bar some of the doors. No one should be admitted to such a hospital. I would claim that the only legal, moral, and prudential justification for involuntary confinement is treatment. This opinion, as you will see, puts me at odds with the United States Federal courts. I believe that the protection of society is and should be the domain of the criminal justice system. I believe that the treatment of the mentally ill should be the domain of the mental health system. The blurring of these two functions is responsible for much that has gone wrong at the intersections between law and psychiatry. The result is that the mental health system typically neither properly protects society nor properly treats patients. At any rate, some Federal courts continue to take the Gault approach: since the public hospitals provide such a shockingly low standard of care, nothing will be lost if we make it harder for patients to get in by imposing procedural safeguards.

The third perspective inspiring legal reform came from a more radical view. It was argued that mental illness was a myth, that psychiatric diagnosis was equivalent to the Spanish Inquisition, that the so-called mentally ill were merely the scapegoats of the dominant social order. Now every American statute on civil commitment has as its first premise the factual empirical assumption that mental illness exists. Absent that premise, and these statutes and all others at the intersection of law and psychiatry are without foundation. Radical antipsychiatrists like Dr Thomas Szasz reject this first premise, and quite consistently favor not only the abolition of civil commitment but also the abolition of the insanity defense and all other statutes, rules of law or regulations premised on the reality of a category of mental illness.

This perspective has deeply influenced legal reform in America, although typically judges make much less straightforward arguments than those of Dr Szasz. Courts concluded that even if there was such a thing as mental illness, psychiatrists could not agree what it was. Nonetheless, the typical legal reforms have retained the requirement of a diagnosis of mental illness, but have emphasized the additional objective requirements necessary for involuntary confinement. One Federal judge, in striking down the medical model of civil commitment, commented that along with his concern that personal freedom was at stake, 'a close second consideration has been that the diagnosis of mental illness leaves too much to subjective choice by less than neutral individuals'.[10] Psychiatry is too unreliable and too subjective; what is needed for civil commitment is an objective legal standard. The objective legal standard is dangerous behavior.

I am prepared to recognize the law's struggle to find a fair moral principle to justify deprivation of liberty. Legal activists found it in John Stuart Mill: 'The only purpose for which power can rightfully be exercised over any member of a civilized community against his will is to prevent harm to others.' This is the rationale for the objective standard of civil libertarians. They have argued that 'dangerous to others' should be the only justification for civil commitment, and the Federal courts, though unwilling to go that far, clearly have aimed in that direction. The sudden popularity of this objective view among legal authorities of all political persuasions was extraordinary. Even under President Nixon and Attorney General Mitchell (neither of whom is remembered as a champion of civil liberties) I was informed by the Justice Department that in their view a finding of dangerousness was constitutionally mandated for civil commitment. When I wrote to the Assistant Attorney General in charge of the civil rights division questioning the wisdom and the constitutional necessity for this view I received a page and a half of irrelevant legal citations – it was a *fait accompli*. It is no longer, by the way; things are changing, and in a few states legislatures have restored medical criteria for confinement.

But it is important to remember why dangerousness seemed like an objective standard to the legal imagination. If one translated dangerousness into the past act requirement as some Federal courts did, then judges needed to place less reliance on psychiatric testimony. The hearing could be more like a criminal trial: did he or didn't he push the Dean? The whole past act due process approach fits comfortably into an established legal tradition. Secondly, if you thought that psychiatric hospitals were not able to give adequate treatment, then why not limit them to the role of controlling dangerous persons? Finally, if you were sympathetic to the view that psychiatric diagnosis which emphasized mental condition was unreliable, then it seemed more objective to emphasize dangerousness and to avoid psychiatric mumbo jumbo. This is the kind of legal thinking that animated reform in the United States.

Unfortunately this is not a sensible basis for deciding who belongs in a mental hospital. The vast majority of persons who have serious mental illness and will benefit from short-term involuntary psychiatric treatment are not dangerous; they are acutely psychotic like the law student Mr X. On the other hand, the vast majority of violence in the United States is caused by people who are not acutely psychotic and who do not benefit from short-term involuntary psychiatric treatment. Thus the standard of dangerousness typically confines people who do not belong in modern psychiatric hospitals geared to rapid treatment of acute conditions.

Secondly, if a person like Mr X had committed a serious act of violence, if he had killed the Dean instead of pushing him, then he would certainly have been prosecuted for murder. Very violent persons are not civilly committed; they are prosecuted in the criminal courts – even if they are, like Hinckley, found not guilty by reason of insanity. It is politically unacceptable not to prosecute the violent insane. Thus, the kind of person civilly committed under the dangerousness standard rarely poses a real threat to society; he is not considered important enough for the criminal justice system. The objective standard does not, in practice, offer real protection to society. It usually, with some notable exceptions, ends up confining chronic troublemakers who commit minor, if repetitive, acts of violence.[11]

Thirdly, psychiatrists unfortunately have no cure for violence, except in those rare instances when it is a symptom of a treatable mental disorder. Nor is there any empirical evidence that we can identify those notable exceptions with serious mental illness who pose a real threat to society (i.e. those who without a past history of violence will become violent). The courts, under their objective standard, are sending patients who cannot be properly identified to hospitals that cannot properly treat them and cannot control them. Indeed, the courts increasingly limit the use of restraint, seclusion, and other controls in mental hospitals.[12]

Fourthly, this method of selecting patients for involuntary confinement is destroying the possibility of treating anyone in our public mental hospitals.[13] When a critical mass of such untreatable and uncontrollable persons is confined in a hospital, chaos results. Recently, there have been reports of increased rates of violence in mental hospitals, including violence against the staff.[14] My own view is that this increase in violence is directly attributable to the new standard of civil commitment: it selects out a population which transforms hospitals into prisons and the medical staff into guards.

Now I have already indicated that very few of these patients are seriously violent, but some are. The question arises: does not the general public at least get some protection by confining them, even if the other patients and the staff still willing to work in these hospitals become the victims of violence? My answer to that is no. Twenty years ago when patients were confined for 13 years the public was protected. Today the entire approach of psychiatry is geared to short-term hospitalization. If psychiatrists could tell which patients would be seriously violent, they could selectively confine them. But the truth is, we cannot. All of these patients are rapidly sent out through the revolving doors. Current legal policy and current mental health policy could not be more in conflict. The result is bad treatment for patients, poor security for the public and bad morale in the public mental health sector. Because it is unfair to confine a person who cannot be treated, because it is harmful to the treatment of other patients, and because it fails to protect the community, the criminalization of civil commitment favored by civil libertarians is a failure.

This failure is compounded by the fact that those with serious mental illness who would benefit from short-term involuntary treatment and are incompetent to make treatment decisions will not be hospitalized. Responsible legislatures have begun to remedy this situation.

During most of this century, psychiatrists in the United States have used civil commitment improperly. They have confined people in hospitals that had neither the ability to treat them nor the resources to provide a humane asylum. Those patients have suffered as a result. Psychiatrists cannot be given – we do not deserve – a free hand in civil commitment. Loss of liberty should be by judicial decision. Involuntary treatment should be by judicial decision. But in establishing the standards for civil commitment and involuntary treatment, an attempt must be found to articulate objective legal criteria for hospitalization – *not* for imprisonment. Elsewhere I have suggested what those hospitalization criteria would be; they include a serious mental illness, evidence that the person is suffering, and is incapable of making competent medical decisions. If these criteria are met, a proxy decision by judge or jury could mandate a specific, time-limited treatment program. Some people meeting these criteria would be classified as dangerous. Most would not, but anyone involuntarily confined in this manner would belong in a place that at last deserved to be called a hospital. The American Psychiatric Association has now offered a model mental health act which includes some of these ideas.[15] It does not solve all of the problems but it is a step in the right direction, the decriminalization of civil commitment. Psychiatrists in Great Britain will recognize that it is a step in the right direction of the approach taken by the British Royal Commission of 1957.

NOTES

1. US Gen. Accounting Office, *Returning the Mentally Disabled to the Community: Government Needs to Do More* (1977).
2. *Bartley* v. *Kremens* 402 F. Supp. 1039 (ED PA 1975).
3. *Lessard* v. *Schmidt* 349 F. Supp. 1078 (ED Wisc. 1972).
4. A.A. Stone, *Law, Psychiatry and Morality* (American Psychiatric Press, Washington, DC, 1984), Chapter II.
5. See for example *Bartley* v. *Kremens*, note 2 above.
6. Stone, note 4 above, Chapter VI.
7. A.B. Hollingshead and F.C. Redlich, *Social Class and Mental Illness: A Community Study* (Wiley, New York, 1958).
8. L. Bellak, *Schizophrenia: A Review of the Syndrome* (Basic Books, New York, 1958), p. 75.
9. Application of Gault 387 US 1 (1967).
10. *Suzuki* v. *Gluisenberg* 411 F. Supp. 1113 (DC Hawaii 1976).
11. Stone, note 4 above, Chapter II.
12. *Rogers* v. *Okin* 478 F. Supp. 1342 (DC Mass. 1979).
13. J.R. Lion, W. Snyder and G.F. Merill, 'Underreporting of assaults on staff in a state hospital', *Hospital and Community Psychiatry*, 32 (1981), 497–8.
14. C.D. Stromberg and A.A. Stone, 'A model state law on civil commitment of the mentally ill', *Harvard Journal of Legislation*, 20 (2) (1983), 275–396.

The recent Mental Health Act in the United Kingdom: issues and perspectives

ROBERT BLUGLASS

The new Mental Health Act for England and Wales which came into force on 30 September 1983 is a landmark in the history of the care of the mentally ill and mentally handicapped. It is of importance for a number of reasons. It is not simply a cosmetic improvement to the generally successful Mental Health Act of 1959, but represents the conclusion of a lengthy period of intense debate reflecting the growing interest and concern for human rights and the continuing commitment of mental health workers to ensure that patients receive the treatment and relief from suffering that they need. The 1959 Act was itself a considerable innovation with its adoption of informal admission procedures, the movement away from judicially approved commitment and the establishment of independent Mental Health Review Tribunals to reconsider compulsorily detained psychiatric patients. Curran (1978), in his comparative analysis of mental health legislation across the world, has demonstrated the extensive imitation of these innovations by many other countries.

The 1959 Act followed a comprehensive review of the law relating to mental illness and 'mental deficiency' by a Royal Commission established during a period of therapeutic optimism and social legislative reform, when the mental health laws of England and Wales were still based upon the accumulated statutes of the nineteenth century and early decades of the twentieth. However, it preceded by several years the international human rights movement that resulted in concentrated activity in North America and in the declarations of human and political rights of the United Nations and other international bodies such as the European Convention on Human Rights. There were specific provisions in relation to the field of mental health in the Declaration of the Rights of the Child adopted by the United Nations in 1959, the Declaration of the Rights of

Mentally Retarded Persons in 1971 and the Declaration of the Rights of Disabled Persons (which includes the physically and mentally incapacitated) in 1977. In North America the courts were used as a forum in which to claim constitutional rights for mental patients (McGarry and Kaplan, 1973) and subsequently reforming legislation was passed by many American states and Canadian provinces. The international declarations and the new reforms of mental health legislation confirmed the principle that disabled persons have the same fundamental rights as their fellow citizens, including a right to treatment.

In England and Wales a developing awareness of the force of the human rights movement, linked with a growing distrust of the mental health professions and medical paternalism, led to a re-evaluation of the 1959 Act by a number of leading professional organisations. The National Association of Mental Health (MIND), an increasingly articulate body, and its Legal Director, also published a series of analytical books and papers pointing to the need for reform (Gostin, 1975, 1977).

All this activity eventually resulted in the central government of the 1970s giving consideration to reforming legislation and ultimately to the introduction of a Mental Health (Amendment) Bill by the Conservative Government in 1981.

The new Mental Health Act (the Mental Health Act 1983) amends the previous legislation with the main objective of improving the rights of patients, but it does not alter the basic structure and philosophy of the 1959 Act. Informal admission, whenever possible, remains the keystone and compulsory detention depends upon an application by the relatives or a trained social worker to the managers of a hospital supported by the medical recommendations of two doctors. There seems to be no doubt that a non-judicial procedure continues to be preferred by patients, who find the involvement of courts or judges in a procedure that is primarily concerned with medical need, inappropriate and distasteful. It is a system preferred by the majority of jurisdictions reviewed by Curran in 1978, but is paradoxically criticised by campaigning groups, sometimes anti-psychiatry in outlook, who continue to express suspicion of the authority and integrity of the medical profession and favour lay or judicial monitoring of commitment procedures.

However, new safeguards against unnecessary or inappropriate commitment are introduced in the new Act. The grounds justifying the detention of a patient are more stringent than before. Both the doctors and the social worker (where the social worker is making the application for admission) must agree that hospital admission is the most appropriate way of managing the case, and where the form of mental disorder is classified as psychopathy or mental impairment, the doctors must have predicted that the condition is treatable. The definition of treatment is a wide one and includes 'nursing and care, habilitation and rehabilitation under medical supervision' (section 145). A subsequent inability to treat the patient might lead to the conclusion that there are no continued grounds to justify detaining him.

In many countries there has been a general trend away from short-term hospitalisation where there is increased opportunity to assess the need for involuntary detention in the community; but despite this, compulsory admission for observation for 28 days has been the most frequently used method of detention (apart from the emergency procedures) in England and Wales from the beginning. Emergency admission continues to be for a period of 72 hours, after which time a longer-term detention order must be invoked, or alternatively, the patient may remain in hospital informally or be allowed to leave. Many countries have reduced the period during which a patient may be detained as an emergency measure, to diminish the stigma to the patient. In this country the changes have been in the time periods during which action must be taken either by those applying to the hospital for the admission of the patient or by the examining doctor. This is to ensure that emergency procedures are used in genuine emergencies, not simply to convenience the doctor, as has appeared to have happened, not uncommonly, in the past.

Previously, many countries allowed an indefinite commitment for care and treatment, but there has been an increasing trend towards an initial limited detention with a periodic review, as provided by the 1959 Act. The initial period was 12 months extendable for a further 12 months and then requiring review at two-yearly intervals. The patient had one opportunity to apply to have his case reviewed by a Tribunal during each of these periods of detention. Under the new Act the periods have been halved, improving the patient's rights and safeguards by requiring a review of his case twice as often as previously and giving twice as many opportunities to apply to a Tribunal. It will be observed that the periods of detention remain substantial in England and Wales, longer than the permitted periods in many other jurisdictions, such as California or Alberta, Canada (30 days); also, the periodic evaluations, although now required by statute to be more detailed, are conducted by the doctor in charge of the case.

In most countries mental health legislation is limited to the controls and rights associated with involuntary hospitalisation. A feature of the legislation in England and Wales, which is possibly unique, is the inclusion of powers to place a mentally disordered person, over the age of 16, under the care of a guardian who may be a named individual, such as a relative or friend, or the local authority providing social services who will delegate the functions of the guardian to a social worker. Previously the powers of guardians were exceptionally wide, allowing total control of the patient as if he were a child; the guardian had the authority of a parent. Under the new legislation the guardian's powers are limited to the extent that is necessary to ensure that the patient lives in a suitable place, attends as required for education, training or treatment, and that access is available for those, such as a doctor or social worker, who need to visit him. There are no powers to give consent to treatment on his behalf or to make any other legal decisions for him. Guardianship, therefore, encourages community care with some control upon the patient's liberty and welfare, but now this control is minimal and, like hospitalisation, requires the recommendation of two doctors and an application based upon the existence of a substantial mental disorder. As for hospital detention, patients are placed under guardianship initially for 6 months and further extension is subject to periodic review, with similar rights of application to a Mental Health Review Tribunal.

In this legislation, as previously, provisions for mentally abnormal offenders are included, allowing a court to make a hospital order as an alternative to any other appropriate penalty where an offender has been found guilty of an offence punishable by imprisonment. Two doctors must give evidence and the effect of such an order is similar to compulsory hospitalisation of a patient from the community, with similar rights of review and application to a Mental Health Review Tribunal. Once committed to hospital the offender is a patient and is outside the control of the criminal justice system. Discharge of the patient is a decision to be taken by the doctor in charge of the case or by a Tribunal and the patient may not be returned to court or be sent to prison. In the past this meant that there was no room for reconsideration or second thoughts, but the new legislation introduces an intermediate stage, recommended by the Butler Committee on Mentally Abnormal Offenders (Home Office, 1975). This intermediate stage is the concept of an 'interim hospital order' (section 38), initially for 12 weeks and renewable at 28-day intervals for up to 6 months, which provides an opportunity for assessing the suitability of the patient for a full hospital order if all goes well. There are also new provisions to allow a patient who is awaiting trial to be remanded to hospital, rather than prison, either for a report on his mental condition or for treatment, if his mental disorder is sufficiently serious to justify it.

The Mental Health Act is based upon a legal classification of mental disorder which includes mental illness but also contains two other categories: psychopathic disorder and two forms of 'arrested or incomplete development of mind', now called 'mental impairment' and 'severe mental impairment'. Psychopathic disorder and these new categories of mental handicap (or mental deficiency or retardation) have been the subject of much debate and disagreement.

Psychopathic disorder was introduced into the previous legislation at a time when many authorities considered that the term referred to a recognisable and definitive form of mental disorder which had its origins in an underlying pathology of the brain which would, in due course, be identified. Even at this time, however, there was much dispute about the appropriateness of the term within the Act, since it appeared simply to describe persistently dangerous or antisocial behaviour, implying that some form of abnormality of mind distinguished the patient from others for whom medical treatment was not suitable. Susceptibility to treatment was, in effect, the justification for making the diagnosis – a curious and circular argument. The definition of psychopathic disorder under the previous Act was, therefore, 'a persistent disorder or disability of mind (whether or not including subnormality of intelligence) which results in abnormally aggressive or seriously irresponsible conduct on the part of the patient and requires, or is susceptible to medical treatment'.

In the years that followed, practitioners became increasingly dissatisfied with this definition and considered that the hypothesis upon which it is based is unproven, the wording is semantically unsatisfactory and unjustified and the term tends to be stigmatic and harmful. Many psychiatrists argue that these patients are basically untreatable and there has been a reduction in the number of patients admitted to hospital with this label in recent years. The Butler Committee comprehensively reviewed the diversity of opinion as to the place of psychopathic disorder or 'personality disorder' within legislation. Although the Committee had no doubt about the widespread dissatisfaction with the category 'psychopathic disorder', they observed that it is one thing to consider introducing it for the first time, but quite a different matter to withdraw it after it has been in a statute for so many years. The Committee tended to favour amending the Act to allow the involuntary committal of individuals suffering from personality disorder (which would not be further defined) where it was in the interests of the patient and the public. They suggested that not all individuals who demonstrated personality disorders were necessarily treatable, but some were, and they should have the benefit of hospital care. For others, particularly offenders, the prison system should be made aware of its responsibility to deal with dangerous and antisocial individuals who did not justify admission to hospital, and it was recommended that special training units be developed within the prison system offering work and activity based upon education and training programmes.

Although the Butler Committee reported in 1975, as with many other recommendations in the Report there has been no progress, or even discussion, on setting up training units, even on an experimental basis. The 1983 Act did, though, go some way towards modifying the law along the lines suggested by Butler. Psychopathic disorder remains one of the categories of mental disorder upon which the Mental Health Act is based, but compulsory admission is now restricted to cases where treatment can be expected 'to alleviate or prevent deterioration'. The committed patient who is suffering from psychopathic disorder will, therefore, have an expectation that he will receive such treatment – one of the basic justifications for his admission. This is also the case with respect to 'mental impairment' and, further in the legislation, for the continued detention, after review, of individuals suffering from mental illness and 'severe mental impairment'. The right to treatment is implied, although not statutorily or constitutionally established, and a failure to provide it adequately could form the basis of an application to a Mental Health Review Tribunal to have detention reconsidered.

The 1959 Mental Health Act included the mentally retarded within its scope. In England and Wales the anxiety to improve the conditions of this group of patients, to elevate their status, and diminish prejudice, has resulted in periodic efforts to seek a new and less pejorative terminology (although cynics have not failed to observe that redefinition is not generally accompanied by an improvement in resources for patient care). The English Act referred to subnormality (and severe subnormality); the Scottish to mental deficiency (now replaced by mental handicap). The justification for including these patients within the scope of mental health legislation was passionately challenged by voluntary groups representing them when the Amendment Bill was proceeding through Parliament. The Government had intended to replace subnormality (in the previous Act) by 'mental handicap', the term that is in general use in the United Kingdom, at the same time redefining the category to stress social as well as intellectual limitation. However, the view was strongly expressed that mental handicap is not a condition which is likely to require involuntary admission to hospital and, furthermore, is a fundamentally different condition to mental illness in that it is a disorder of social functioning and not an illness. It should not be confused with disorders such as schizophrenia and dementia. Yet it was eventually conceded that a minority of handicapped individuals do sometimes require committal to hospital because of their behaviour and for their own or others' benefit. To distinguish this group from the rest the Government created a new category which it termed 'mental impairment', a classification applying only to mentally handicapped patients who exhibit abnormally aggressive or seriously irresponsible conduct. Only this group could be considered for involuntary admission or guardianship. Other mentally handicapped patients are only liable to be detained for very short periods and only for assessment.

This is a novel way of meeting the criticisms of the charities, but it may lead to new problems in the management and treatment of mentally handicapped patients who do not show 'abnormally aggressive or seriously irresponsible conduct' but refuse treatment, or are very unco-operative and difficult to manage. Insufficient thought has been given to the problems that may arise, such as consent to treatment and control of difficult mentally handicapped patients.

The thrust of the new legislation and the repeated concern of Members of Parliament was to encourage community care wherever possible and confine hospital care, particularly involuntary admission, to a restricted group for whom it is the only alternative. Although the medical profession would not dispute the wisdom of this policy, the vast majority of doctors have, with their non-medical colleagues, been pursuing this aim for many years. Indeed, the psychiatrists were responsible in the United Kingdom for promoting the open-door policy, fostering the notion of community care, of day hospitals, community-based psychiatrists and many other similar developments, partly made possible by concurrent developments in psychopharmacology and improved staffing. Despite this progress, the notion of care in the community has not been met by an increased provision of residential accommodation, hostels, trained social workers, community nurses or community care teams, many of which it is the responsibility not of the health authorities, but of local authorities to provide.

There has often been little alternative to hospital care, which in some cases has provided 'asylum' for the patient in the true sense. Yet doctors have been aware that they alone are accused of failing in their responsibility to keep patients in the community and that the interests of the patient are deemed to have been subordinated to the whims of an over-restrictive and conservative profession, paternalistic in attitude, insufficiently aware of the rights of patients and hostile to the demands of consumerism. The criticism does not appear to have been voiced by the patients themselves in substantial numbers, but is heard from the highly specialised civil rights groups, from the increasingly competitive paramedical professions and in Parliament from its Members in both Houses. A depressing element in the debates associated with the amending legislation was often the anti-psychiatric, indeed, anti-medical, views expressed which seemed to reflect a lack of confidence in professional expertise and clinical judgment, and support for 'common sense' and defensive mechanisms to protect the patient. Although much of this is unfair, it must be taken seriously and indeed has had to be faced squarely by the psychiatrists' professional body, the Royal College of Psychiatrists. Psychiatrists have for some considerable time been engaged in the examination of forms of medical audit or peer review, public education and the need for an independent body, analogous to the pre-1959 Board of Control, to protect the rights of patients and the legal position of staff caring for them.

The need to control the activities and clinical freedom of the medical profession which is, to a considerable extent, reflected in the new legislation and was expressed often vehemently in the Parliamentary debates, must eventually be accepted by doctors and without a paranoid reaction of rejection. It is symptomatic of a much more extensive disenchantment with conventional methods of health care which has led to a movement towards alternative medicine, and the creation of the British Holistic Medical Association, a degree course in alternative medicine at the Polytechnic of Central London, and in the United States the establishment of bodies such as the Esslin Institute in California. *The Times* in a leading article on 10 August 1983, suggested that people are 'groping for some extra dimension to health care, which goes beyond a state of dissatisfaction with hospital waiting lists and crowded clinics'. It suggests that many more people now are coming to 'reject the purely scientific approach to medicine' while the medical establishment 'continues to disregard the personal factor in medicine'. Clearly those of us with a responsibility for the education of doctors must consider how this challenge should be met.

However, there were many parliamentarians who were determined to press for better community care and recognised that legislation alone cannot change the quality of life for patients but can only facilitate ways of improving it. Despite Government resistance, a statutory duty was introduced into the Act which places an obligation on local authorities to provide aftercare for discharged detained patients, even though already required by several Acts of Parliament; but this did not mean any additional funding to provide it.

The most important innovation is probably the establishment of an independent Commission, a multidisciplinary body with lay membership, and including lawyers, which has the responsibility for protecting the rights of individual detained patients. The Commission has about ninety members who monitor admission procedures, deal with complaints, inspect professional practices and standards in all psychiatric hospitals, will establish a Code of Practice and will provide independent second medical opinions, to operate the new consent to treatment procedures. The Mental Health Act Commission is an alternative to patients' advisors, legal officers in hospital or the involvement of courts for the protection of the patient.

The Mental Health Act 1983 also, for the first time, defines the grounds for treating patients without consent. It was previously assumed that if a patient was detained for treatment (section 26, Mental Health Act 1959) then such treatment as may be necessary could be administered irrespective of the patient's wishes and those of the relatives. This view was endorsed by the Department of Health and Social Security on several occasions (e.g. Butler Committee Report, p. 51). However, the presumption of 'global incompetence' as Alan Stone has termed it (Stone, 1981) was increasingly challenged by MIND (Gostin, 1981) and others, as it had been in the United States. The Act now recognises that involuntary admission does not necessarily imply incompetence. Competency is a matter to be considered separately, when it is proposed to offer forms of treatment to the patient. It was, therefore, necessary to devise procedures to determine competency after commitment, and an acceptable authority to allow treatment to be given to those who are incompetent.

Many jurisdictions provide that incompetence should be determined by a judge. The medical profession in the United Kingdom argued strongly that the doctor–patient relationship is at the heart of treatment decisions and that the determination of competency is an important element of such decision-making. Even Ian Kennedy (1978), who is not noted for his support of the medical establishment, has commented that 'a legal system which sees the contact of a doctor with his patient as an assault or battery made lawful by consent, and which rests on the notion of informed consent, without showing any real understanding of the dynamics of the doctor–patient relationship, is in danger of losing respect'.

These arguments were accepted by the Government and the new legislation provides several levels of control. 'Serious' treatments, psychosurgery and the surgical implantation of hormones to reduce male sexual drive, may not be given to any patient, detained or informal, inpatient or outpatient, unless (*a*) the patient consents, (*b*) a medical and two non-medical assessors have agreed that the patient is competent to consent and (c) the doctor, after consulting members of the treatment team has agreed that the treatment is justified in the particular case. Other treatments can be added to this group in the future.

Secondly, electroconvulsive therapy and, after the first 3 months of administration, any medicines, may not be given to a detained patient for the treatment of mental disorder without the patient's informed consent. However, if he is thought to be incompetent to consent, or his consent is irrationally refused, the treatment may be given if it is supported by an independent second medical opinion provided by a medical commissioner or a doctor appointed for the purpose. Other treatments may be added to this list.

There are provisions dealing with a plan of treatment, involving several medicines for instance, with withdrawal of consent and with emergency treatment.

The introduction into English law of a statutory test of competence to consent for psychiatric patients (that the patient is capable of understanding the nature, purpose and likely effects of the treatment) must raise the question as to what implications this has for voluntary or informal patients suffering not only from psychiatric disorder but also from physical illness. If the detained psychiatric patient now has a statutory right to consent if competent, and competence is defined, this standard must surely extend before long to all other patients. Is it not only a matter of time before the statutory certification of competence for detained psychiatric patients becomes a requirement for all other patients, and should this not be the case?

The new requirements suggest other anomalies. The need to demonstrate competence is limited to treatments given for mental disorder. There is no authority to treat physical illness in the same patient, despite his refusal or incompetency to consent. Further, what is the future position of non-detained mentally handicapped patients and the confused or demented elderly? The introduction of statutory procedures to overrule detained patients implies that others (except in emergencies) may only be treated with their informed consent. How should doctors be advised to proceed?

Probably as long as we remain, happily, not a very litigious community, doctors will work out these problems with patients and relatives in a common-sense way, in their patients' best interests. However, if there should be any substantial increase in medical malpractice litigation, as has occurred in the United States, then there will be considerable problems and a move to defensive medicine. It is very much to be hoped that this can be avoided.

Those of us who have been intimately involved in the shaping of the new Mental Health Act feel inevitably optimistic that it will be successful. In many ways it marks the beginning of a new era and we may hope that, with half an eye on other legal systems, we have avoided an over-legalistic approach and that we will be able to sustain, or even enhance, the reputation of the Act of 1959.

REFERENCES

Bluglass, R. (1983). *A Guide to the Mental Health Act 1983.* Churchill Livingstone, London and Edinburgh. [For a detailed review of the 1983 Act.]

Curran, W.J. (1978). Comparative analysis of mental health legislation in forty-three countries: a discussion of historical trends. *International Journal of Law and Psychiatry*, 1, 79–92.

Gostin, L.O. (1975, 1977). *A Human Condition*, vols. 1 and 2. National Association of Mental Health, London.

Gostin, L.O. (1981). Observations on consent to treatment and review of clinical judgment in psychiatry: a discussion paper. *Journal of the Royal Society of Medicine*, 74, 742–52.

Home Office, DHSS and Welsh Office (1975). *Report of the Committee on Mentally Abnormal Offenders* (Butler Committee). Command 6244. HMSO, London.

Kennedy, I. (1978). The law relating to the treatment of the terminally ill. In *The Management of Terminal Disease*, ed. C.M. Saunders. Edward Arnold, London.

McGarry, A.L. and Kaplan, H.A. (1973). Overview: current trends in mental health law. *American Journal of Psychiatry*, 130, 521.

Stone, A. (1981). The right to refuse treatment. *Archives of General Psychiatry*, 38, 358–62.

Medical and social consequences of the Italian Psychiatric Care Act of 1978

P. SARTESCHI, G.B. CASSANO, M. MAURI and
A. PETRACCA

Introduction

A wide-ranging debate over psychiatric care in general and the Psychiatric Care Act of 1978 in particular, has been going on at various levels of Italian society. Laymen have been expressing their views in favour of 'open' or 'closed' mental hospitals; journalists have been surveying public opinion on the question, and presenting the opinions of different sides; and psychiatrists and politicians have been tirelessly bringing forward arguments about the applicability and feasibility of the new law. Before the 1978 Act, psychiatric care in Italy had been marked by a long period of legislative inertia going back to Act 36 of 1904, which largely reflected the psychiatric legislation of other European countries. Considering the year in which it was passed, the 1904 Act was effective and commendable. It permitted the founding of new psychiatric hospitals and laid down regulations for compulsory admission. This law, however, belonged to the pretherapeutic era of psychiatry and the impact of psychopharmacology quickly made it out of date. The major shortcoming of the 1904 Act was that it lasted too long and almost exclusively provided for the admission of patients without considering how their discharge was to be achieved. Only in 1968 was the 1904 Act partly updated by the addition of article 4, which provided for voluntary admission to psychiatric institutions and for the founding of mental health centres for patients discharged from psychiatric hospitals.

The 1904 Act, which is still harshly criticized because of the falsely apocalyptic way it has been presented by the 'new psychiatry' as the law of strait-jackets, of electroconvulsive therapy, and of total institutionalization, was based upon a fundamental concept which has been too readily discarded: that of dangerousness to oneself and to others. Conversely, the new psychiatry based its approach on the assumption that mental illness is the result of a distortion in the communication network set up between the individual and his family, his work environment and society in general.

Ideological pressures in the late sixties and seventies, the objective and urgent need for a soundly based approach to the problem, and indecisiveness and clashes in Parliament and in political parties, came together to bring the issue of a change in the law on psychiatric care to a stalemate overcharged with tension. In this situation the Italian Radical Party called for a referendum to abolish mental hospitals through the abrogation of the 1904 Act. To forestall this, the main political parties were forced to come to an agreement. Thus, the bill, known in Italy by its number, 180, went through parliament very quickly, and became the new tool for the provision of psychiatric care. This law was later included, unchanged, in Act 833, which laid the foundations of the Italian National Health System.

The passing of this law certainly meant that an opportunity had been lost; the preceding period had seen the gradual development of a different concept of mental illness that was not tied to any specific ideological position, and allowed for the integration of somatic-biological psychiatry with the latest trends in social psychiatry. The abrupt change in the situation brought about by the 1978 Act has resulted in the replacement of the old model of psychiatric care with a new one, which has even more rigid and absolutely dominant characteristics. This situation has its historical precedents. Even in the last decade of the nineteenth century the issue of mental institutions, that is, of inpatient treatment versus community care based on outpatient treatment, divided the medical world. Andrea Verga, an Italian psychiatrist, formulated the following query in 1897: 'is it more logical and convenient to treat someone who is mentally ill within his family or in those places which the advancement of society and science has prepared and which are called mental hospitals?' It may be worth mentioning that at that time the opponents of mental hospitals included the most conservative classes, such as the clergy.

It is likely that a more thoughtful approach to reform of the 1904 Act would have led to less disruption, and would gradually have fostered a more outpatient-centred form of psychiatric care without sacrificing an all-round view of patient needs and psychiatry's many facets.

Distinctive features of the Act

In the 1978 Act an attempt was undoubtedly made to deal with the major problems raised by psychiatric care by laying down a series of innovative principles:

1. Any distinction between mental illnesses and other diseases is to be abolished, so eliminating the notion of the dangerousness of psychiatric patients.

2. Even for psychiatric patients 'health survey and treatment are voluntary' (art. 33, para. 1).

3. Article 2 states that there should be a shift of patient care towards outpatient services by limiting the number and length of inpatient treatments. Regulation at regional level was, in fact, supposed to allow for the setting up of 'territorial outpatient Services and Units within the local Health Unit' (Legge, 1978) to provide 'prevention, care, and rehabilitation for mental disorders' (art. 34, paras. 1–3).

4. Compulsory treatment (C.T.) should be 'performed by public territorial health services and units' (art. 3, para. 4), but the admission (to small inpatient units within general hospitals) is warranted 'only if mental disorders are such that urgent therapeutic measures are needed, if these are not accepted by the patient and if there are no conditions or circumstances that allow the adoption of rapid and effective outpatient medical measures' (art. 34, para. 4). Moreover, C.T. 'must be accompanied by initiatives which aim to assure the consent and participation of the patient' (art. 33, para. 5). In order to reduce the frequency of C.T., 'initiatives for prevention and medical education' (art. 33, para. 5) should be taken. C.T. must be authorized by the Mayor after a proposal to this effect has been made by a physician; in the case of inpatient treatment, this has to be countersigned by a doctor working for the local Health System. Within 48 hours the Tutelary Judge must be informed, in order to ratify C.T. during the next 48 hours. C.T. authorization may be given for a maximum of 7 days; whenever a longer period of inpatient care is needed, the doctor responsible for the Psychiatric Service of the Local Health Authority has to make a proposal to the Mayor, who will inform the Tutelary Judge, in line with the procedure mentioned above. There is also provision for the revocation or modification of a C.T. order through a legal request to be made to the Mayor or the Tribunal.

5. C.T. also has to take place 'inside general hospitals, at specific psychiatric Units for diagnosis and treatment, and these must be connected with outpatient Services and Units so that therapeutic continuity is ensured'. The number of beds within such psychiatric inpatient Units is established by the Regional Health Plan (art. 34, para. 5).

6. Article 64 says that the Region has to bring about 'the gradual elimination of Mental Hospitals' by not allowing any new admissions and by prohibiting the 'building of new Mental Hospitals, the use of those in

existence as the psychiatric wards of general hospitals, and the setting up within general hospitals of psychiatric wards or neurological or neuropsychiatric Units'.

Ideological background and objective of the Act

The ideological background of the 1978 Act was very simple and schematic: firstly, mental disturbances were supposed to spring from the violence produced by society, and secondly the mentally ill were supposed to be the object of repression, which turned them into social outcasts. In this process mental hospitals were viewed as playing a major role in producing the repression and social rejection of the mentally ill, as well as the disorders typical of institutionalization. The refusal of any traditional nosography and thus of any means of treatment was the result of the prejudice that 'psychiatric cases' were simply the result of exclusion and institutionalization.

It may be recalled that some centres, even in the last few years, have refused to adopt an adequate diagnostic approach since this might represent 'another means of turning the patient into an outcast'. In such centres no valid epidemiological studies have been performed and most of the efforts made have been devoted to trying to solve patients' social problems, while the psychopathological picture has been overlooked. An attitude of this kind spread quickly through the mass media to the people and was strongly supported by trade unions, the student movement and most political parties.

In Italy as in other western countries, a sharp fall in the number of people staying in mental hospitals had taken place between 1960 and 1978, but the 1978 Act, in accordance with the ideology mentioned above, laid down that mental hospitals and other institutions for the mentally ill should be immediately abolished, so expressing a real phobia towards any structure which might induce institutionalization.

The Italian Members of Parliament who passed the law were worried about the perverse effects any kind of 'total institution might leave on patients, seeing such effects as a source of suffering and adaptive behaviour leading to more psychiatric symptoms'. Their first reaction was to make it illegal to use any of the mental hospitals existing in 1978 or to build any new institution for the long-term treatment of mental patients. Secondly, Members were worried that any kind of psychiatric institution, even those which were an alternative to mental hospitals, might become antitherapeutic. The law that was passed thus did not allow for any organized structure to replace the old psychiatric system.

More specifically, the 1978 Act intended to:

1. Bring about the closure of psychiatric hospitals, and supersede a system based on constraint and control.
2. Create decentralized community structures for the prevention of mental illness, and for the treatment and rehabilitation of psychiatric patients.
3. Accord priority to voluntary psychiatric treatment over the compulsory approach.
4. Eliminate the fragmentation of the interventions, and promote a so-called global answer to psychiatric disturbances, through a pivotal role of an extra-hospital service.

The Act called for the prevention, treatment and rehabilitation of mental illness outside the hospital milieu. In it, regional governments are called upon to draw up and coordinate a programme for psychiatric care and the promotion of mental health in cooperation with all other health and medical structures.

Thus, after the Act's radical interruption of the functioning of the previous hospitals, it left most of the area of mental health to the imagination and fantasy of local administrators, who were expected to adopt a model of therapeutic continuity springing from sector psychiatry that was to be put into practice by a team operating both in small inpatient psychiatric wards and in the community. Besides this, the problem of alternative institutions such as day and night hospitals, family homes, homes for the elderly and protected workshops remains completely unsolved.

Medical and social consequences of the Act

The new law completely disoriented physicians and psychiatrists; there was a sudden disruption of the previous system of psychiatric care and this resulted in severe delays in the organization of new psychiatric services. A reform of this kind was bound to be a failure, because of the high dose of populistic optimism that required people to believe that in the absence of adequate inpatient and outpatient services or specialized personnel, an adequate mental health organization could be set up. So far no programme has been devised for the reintegration of the patient into the social milieu, and this vital point has been left to improvisation and uncoordinated dabbling, or, still worse, to the individual theories of medical and paramedical personnel who have not been 'retrained' and who are confronted with the ill-defined concept of the 'community'.

One essential condition for any change in the traditional approach to psychiatry has been completely overlooked; that is the need for specially trained high-level personnel, capable of developing a more complex and varied range of therapeutic responses. Generally, the only change has been the transfer of personnel from psychiatric hospitals to the new services, while the major qualitative differences between these two therapeutic approaches have been ignored. Moreover the diagnostic and therapeutic approach has been seriously undervalued; this has led to undue heterogeneity and to a fall in psychiatric standards in the management of the patient during the early phase of survey and treatment.

A major risk which can be foreseen is the possible evolution of this attitude with regard to the future of patients. The lack of a correct diagnostic approach and of effective treatment will contribute to a progressive increase in chronic patients, especially severe psychotic cases, so creating once again a need for institutions and long-term inpatient treatment and completing a vicious circle that progress in psychiatry had led us to imagine had been definitively broken.

Now, five years after the 1978 Act became law, and after its inclusion within Act 833 (as articles 33, 34 and 35), it may be asserted not only that none of the objectives of this law has been attained, but that there has actually been a severe decline in the quality of psychiatric care, with very unfortunate consequences for patients, their families and society in general. Most of the consequences of the 1978 Act cannot be assessed, because of the lack of reliable data on existing structures, the planning of new ones, the number of voluntary and compulsory admissions, the type of care available in different areas, and the measures taken to assess the efficiency of the various services. So far the planning of studies devoted to collecting and evaluating this type of information has always been delayed, both for organizational reasons and because no clear indication of government policy has been forthcoming. As a result, what information is available is often fragmentary, anecdotal and liable to ambiguous interpetation.

Some data, however, have been ascertained; since 1978, for instance, the number of patients who are currently in a state of restraint in criminal mental asylums has greatly increased, as has the number of admissions to private psychiatric institutes and the percentage of psychiatric patients in private nursing homes for the elderly. An example which might be quoted is that of the 700 residents of an old people's home near Pisa; of these, 40% are patients who have been discharged from mental hospitals in the area and a total of almost 90% have been labelled as psychiatric patients.

Among the most controversial data are those concerning the number of compulsory admissions and the length of inpatient treatment; in fact, such data not only vary from one area to another, but are interpreted in a number of different ways according to the ideological viewpoint of the observer. Thus, a small number of compulsory admissions has often been interpreted as a measure of the efficiency of a particular service, while in fact a desire on the part of the service's staff to appear as efficient as possible may well be the direct cause of a fall in the number of such admissions, given the staff's awareness of the applications of this criterion. Moreover, the same problem may arise over the length of stay in inpatient services, though it seems reasonable to suppose that inpatient treatment lasting an average of 8 days is insufficient for the treatment of a patient suffering from an acute, severe psychiatric condition.

Some of the consequences of the law can be summarized in terms of its repercussions on the various structures and components of society. 'Closed' mental hospitals have had to face an awkward situation: though they should be completely dismantled, they still hold 35000 patients. The outcome is that these patients are left almost entirely to themselves; there is no longer any provision for specialized treatment, there are no psychologists or social workers acting to help them, and no attempts are being made to provide for a programme of rehabilitation and socialization. In many hospitals only one doctor is on night call, and his time is devoted exclusively to coping with medical emergencies. The buildings themselves are not maintained, and no funds are available for even the most obvious necessities. What is more, the number of those living in these mental hospitals is probably higher than the official estimates because of two stratagems. First, some of the patients still living in the hospitals are called 'guests' and are housed in what are called 'protected' apartments. Second, some of the wards have been renamed nursing homes for the elderly; in this way all the psychiatric patients over 65 years of age can be 'recycled' as geriatric patients.

A side-effect of the prohibition against using and building mental hospitals has been a ban on other institutions such as homes for old people or neuropsychiatric units for children. This has taken the form of refusing admission to the existing institutions or slowing down plans for new ones.

Another drawback of the present law is that there is no provision for any type of structure specifically devoted to the care of patients suffering from organic brain syndromes who used to be housed in mental hospitals. This situation sprang from the false assumption that psychiatry within the community could solve every problem; the idea was that a community service could constitute an effective way of identifying and solving the aetiological causes of mental illness, which were considered to be mainly due to environmental factors. No treatment wards would be needed. This has turned out to be incorrect not only with regard to obviously chronic patients, such as severely brain-damaged children or senile patients, but also for those suffering from recurrent psychotic episodes or affective disorders that do not respond to treatment. Most of these patients, therefore, for whom the 1978 Act makes no provision whatsoever, have been simply transferred from mental hospitals to nursing homes or private institutions where, apparently, they are just kept under observation, and often receive very little psychiatric treatment.

A number of patients who had been discharged from mental hospitals and did not succeed in being reintegrated in the social structures they were sent back to, have been 'readmitted' to forensic hospitals, after having committed an offence. Other patients often stay three months or more in University Psychiatric Institutes (which, incidentally, are not even mentioned in the 1978 Act) or in the Diagnosis and Care Psychiatric Services (DCPS), and are often discharged and readmitted frequently, so presenting a 'revolving door' syndrome. *Ad hoc* structures have been formed such as private therapeutic communes, which have been set up particularly to help drug addicts and alcoholics, and premises in private apartments rented by former psychiatric nurses to house discharged psychiatric patients. Other patients, who really need long-term inpatient treatment, have just been sent out to fend for themselves in society and can often be seen living in railway stations or sleeping in public parks or in the fields on the outskirts of towns, so aggravating a feeling of hostility in the population that had supposedly disappeared during the libertarian post-1968 era. All other patients of this type have been sent back to the community, which means that, at best, they have been given back to their families, who now have to face the problem of changing their lives to cope with a mentally disturbed member. In such families it is often a mother, wife or daughter who has to look after the patient, and must thus resume a subordinate role from which she had struggled hard to free herself.

So the situation has become explosive, and some 30 000 families have formed associations (such as ARAP and DIAPSIGRA) which have sought to promote the development of outpatient structures of various types, along with institutions for the hospitalization of severely and chronically ill persons.

The lack of any adequate plan to set up all necessary outpatient services, together with the absence of any provision in the law for their funding, has produced an absolutely chaotic situation at local level. Local psychiatric services do not, in fact, cover the whole country, and the planning of their future development is based upon epidemiological data that are often misleading, and imprecisely collected. The regional governments are autonomously defining what is to be done, often without any coordination or soundly scientifically based knowledge of the situation. Thus what is actually happening is that the only services which have retained a certain efficiency are units similar to the old mental health centres, which, however, are usually only open during office hours; they are understaffed and are overwhelmed by requests for financial support from patients dismissed from mental hospitals. A great deal of effort is wasted in bureaucratic procedures.

Of course, no one doubts the validity of an approach that is specifically organized for certain types of patient, so allowing differentiation between the therapeutic methodologies provided for different categories of patients. Nevertheless, in the DCPS no separation is made between voluntary and compulsory inpatients, so that no specific section is dedicated to compulsorily admitted patients. Moreover, too many psychiatric patients have to be admitted, and they then stay for too short a period. As a result, they may receive too little attention, and in most cases they are discharged with a prescription for a long-acting neuroleptic drug.

As far as the increased risk of violence is concerned, it is difficult to give a comparative evaluation of the figures of hetero- and autoaggressive actions committed by psychiatric patients before and after the new law, and of the possible fall in patients' life span. It is virtually impossible to gather reliable data from personal or local observations of groups of former mental hospital patients or newspaper reports. What is certain is that there is now a fairly frequent phenomenon of psychiatric family members who are killed by their relatives (Censis, 1982).

The potential users of the mental hospitals may be divided approximately into two main categories. The first consists of subjects admitted to and treated in mental hospitals before the 1978 Act came into force; some of these are still in mental hospitals, making up the residual psychiatric group, some are in other institutions such as old people's homes or forensic hospitals, while a few have been assigned to their families or to alternative community structures. The second category consists of those subjects who need long-term treatment that cannot be provided in the community or in wards for acute patients. These patients now live in a precarious equilibrium within their families, and are mostly protected by their relatives; their ages range between 20 and 40 years. This equilibrium may be suddenly upset by the death or illness of their relatives.

Conclusions

The ambitious aim of the Italian Psychiatric Care Act of 1978 was that of founding a mental health service outside hospitals, with a well-established centrality with respect to other intermediate structures. On this basis mental hospitals, as well as other institutions acting as so-called discharge containers for psychiatric patients, were to be scheduled for closure or non-authorization.

Even in the most socially and economically advanced regions of Italy, this model could not be concretely implemented. In regions such as Lombardy, the community health services, which coordinate prevention, treatment and rehabilitation over a large geographic area, include various structures such as DCPS for acute inpatients in general hospitals, residential institutes for resocialization, foster houses and day hospitals. Each of them has been set specific and limited spheres of influence such as admission, resocialization, outpatient treatment, keeping patients within the community, or treatment for chronic patients. This subdivision of the work to be done reflects the extreme difficulties to be met by any attempt to attain the goal of providing a centralized service independent of the inpatient services, in accordance with the aims of the 1978 Act. Again, the inpatient units are central with respect to outpatient services. Within existing residential structures, small new psychiatric hospitals are being created, which appear to be 'discharge containers' very similar to the old mental hospitals.

The need for innovative reform in psychiatric care was particularly urgent in Italy. Legislation had lagged behind the daily activity of psychiatrists and personnel working in the psychiatric field, partly because mental hospitals, especially in Northern Italy, were already implementing an 'open-door' policy. Moreover, their administration had been changed from a pyramidal to a horizontal one, so allowing for a more independent and differentiated approach to patient care. So there was a general expectation that any new law would have followed this trend; but one of the basic objectives of the 1978 Act was that of attempting a particular kind of psychiatric reform, while forestalling the continuance or the creation of institutional structures that had been set up in other countries.

Despite the difficulties that have arisen, a considerable effort is still being made to fulfil the aims of the law, and to avoid the creation of the 'discharge containers' which are so often the end-result of the psychiatric circuit. It must be said that there was initially a naive presumption of success where other countries had failed. Great difficulties are still being experienced in the management of chronic patients and in devising a differentiated approach to acute cases. A global approach appears to be as hard to attain in psychiatry as in all other branches of medicine and, in any case, such an approach may only be possible over a limited sector of psychopathology.

One major need is for modern techniques to be applied in collaboration with specialized scientific centres. On the other hand the value of a continuing link between community psychiatric centres and family doctors should not be underestimated since general practitioners have a special role to play in primary care medicine.

Proposals have now been put forward at various levels for changes to be made in the 1978 Act, and we can hope that, with the institution of a new and better-balanced legislative framework based upon a clear and pragmatic view of mental illness, the foundation will be laid for the development of a truly scientific and humane approach to psychiatric care.

REFERENCES

Censis (1982). *Rapporto sull'assistenza psichiatrica*. Paoline.
Legge 13 Maggio 1978, n. 180. Accertamenti e trattamenti sanitari volontari e obbligatori. *Gazzetta Ufficiale della Repubblica Italiana.*
Pizzi, A. (1978). *Malattie mentali e trattamenti sanitari*. Giuffré, Milan.
Pancheri, P. (1982). La legge '180' e la crisi dell'assistenza psichiatrica. *Medicina*, 1. UTET.
Verga, A. (1897). *Studi anatomici, psicologici e freniatrici*. Manini Wijet, Milan.

Lessons for the future drawn from United States legislation and experience

ROBERT J. CAMPBELL

Forensic psychiatry developed largely in relation to lawyers' efforts to save their clients from a death sentence and involved proving 'facts' about insanity, intent, competence, and the like. It spread to include other facts, such as paternity, the cause of death, and a broad range of data relevant to assessing the presence or extent of malpractice. As all clinicians know, however, what is defined as malpractice has mushroomed in recent years and the umbrella of forensic psychiatry now embraces a considerably larger area than it did even a decade ago.

The essentials of classic forensic psychiatry were the assessment and treatment of those who had been statutorily labeled as dangerous, the protection of the public, and the protection of the rights of patients (including their right to treatment). In a technological society such as ours, however, the roles of medical professionals have become increasingly intertwined with those of legal professionals, for scientific advances in medicine relate more and more to the quality of life and the fundamental rights of individuals, and they raise questions about the effects of interventions in the lives of today's patients on tomorrow's society (Harrison, 1983). At the present time, the phrase 'health law' is used to emphasize the expanded interface between medicine and the law and the substantial body of law that now governs the relations between health care providers, professionals, third-party payers, and patients (Stromberg, 1983).

At first glance, medicine and the other sciences would seem to be a world apart from politics. Closer inspection reveals that, in fact, they have been warily courting each other for centuries. It was in 1859 that Darwin published his monumental work *On the Origin of Species by Means of Natural Selection, or the Preservation of Favoured Races in the Struggle for Life.* Darwin viewed survival as a measure of fitness, and progress as a result of natural selection, exercised through competition. The key to social progress according to some social Darwinists was control of the unfit, which would then provide the answer to poverty, crime, mental illness, mental defect, epilepsy, and a host of social ills.

It would be unfair to suggest that the road to social control was used only by politicians. 'Enlightened' scientists, in reciprocal fashion, sought help from politicians to encourage society to conform with the best health principles of their day, just as in our day we have our advocates of low cholesterol diets and jogging and vitamin C, our opponents of tobacco, alcohol and coffee. Indeed, the whole field of public health depends upon such interrelationship between medicine and politics.

By the 1970s, however, at least in the United States, legislators and other policy-makers had become almost too eager to translate medicine's 'what if's' and 'maybe's' into rules and certainties. During that decade, they passed more laws affecting medicine than in all of the country's history prior to 1965. Now, in the 1980s, approximately 6000 legislative bills pertaining to health are introduced each year in our House of Representatives, and close to 2500 in the Senate.

In wondering where all this might end, some warned long ago that lawyers, not doctors, would be defining the range of treatments that can be used with patients; that lawyers would be setting the criteria and standards by which the doctor chooses from the treatments allowed; that lawyers would be establishing the priorities that must be assigned to different patients. It might have been predicted that psychiatry would be more directly affected than most other medical specialities, for the psychiatrist, because of his general societal functions, is typically entangled in such issues even though by all logic they fall well outside his domain. In the United States in the days before abortion became legally acceptable, it was the psychiatrist who most often was called upon to determine whether an abortion was medically necessary to preserve the sanity or the life of the pregnant woman. It is amazing how few lives and minds seem now to be jeopardized by that same condition, and it has thus – fortunately – become an area where psychiatry feels no particular need to pander to the social pressures of the moment.

Nowadays, the problem is more likely to be one of supporting the paternalistic decisions of other medical specialists. If a patient will not readily submit to his surgeon's or oncologist's recommendation, the psychiatrist may be called upon to support the contention that, *ipso facto*, any such patient must be deranged.

It would be a mistake, I believe, to view the many changes in mental health law and regulations only in terms of the criminal code, criminal responsibility and competence for culpability, the insanity defense, involuntary hospitalization, commitment, detention, and the other specifics in which we recurrently become entangled. They must instead be viewed as part of the larger picture of broad social changes taking place within the United States, and elsewhere, that would ultimately be manifested in a set of responses that I shall call 'consumerism'.

The first psychiatric revolution

Eighteenth-century European reforms brought drastic changes in the humanitarian aspects of confinement of the mentally ill. During that period the overall concern for social change and social progress gave rise to a wave of optimism about the perfectibility of man and his social order. That optimism extended to mental illness and expanded into the first psychiatric revolution. The programs of the 'asylum' that came to be known as 'moral treatment' in the 1840s were widely and extravagantly proclaimed. By 1870, however, those institutions had suffered a dramatic decline from reform to custodial establishments and it was clear that the optimism of the founding reformers rested on a flimsy base.

Since its inception in 1906, the mental hygiene movement in the United States has continued to advocate a preventive approach that, except for birth control, remains still to be invented in the mental health field. One of the assumptions of the preventive approach is that maladaptation in the adult is a result of idiosyncratic experiences in early life, and that true prevention is to be achieved by dispensing enough psychotherapy and enough knowledge of psychodynamics to the parents and educators who shape or influence childhood development. The same logic states that, given any indication of pathology, the earlier the person at risk is identified, the more effective will treatment measures be. Two generations of American parents have already been cowed into submission by psychiatric sleuths uncovering the mistakes Mother made in rearing a Johnny who can't read, and a Portnoy who can't love.

Of course, giving that amount of psychotherapy and dispensing that much knowledge to parents and educators was a massive task. There was so much to be done, and so few people to do it, that it seemed only logical to involve more people and train them to be highly skilled in discrete part-functions. The multiple and changing needs of patients could thereby be met, and the move away from the parochialism of clinical psychiatry would insure a more appropriate dissemination of the new truth. In the midst of all this spreading of the gospel World War II came along, and its avalanche of psychiatric casualties intensified the search for 'stand-ins' or 'extenders' for physicians. As they were found, and trained to perform all those tasks that did not specifically require medical training, they assumed greater responsibility and independence.

The second psychiatric revolution

Once the war was over, many psychiatrists were inclined to pursue a direction different from the one they had taken previously. Some, disenchanted by the inability of their dynamic insights to contain the major mental disorders that had confronted them in the armed forces, tried to move closer to the rest of medicine. Although the actual discoveries of psychopharmacologic agents were largely serendipitous, it was this group of psychiatrists that ultimately built those discoveries into what was called the second psychiatric revolution, the era of psychopharmacology.

Others, under the spell of their exposure to other disciplines and systems, seized the opportunity to pay attention to something other than the doctor–patient relationship and to scrutinize the needs of society. They expanded their horizons and embraced a social and cultural orientation that was well outside the medical model. More and more of the human condition became grist for the interpretative mill and the individual patient came to be understood in terms of cultural or societal forces rather than in terms of symptoms, syndromes and illnesses. Indeed, it became quite unfashionable to speak of nosology and diagnosis, as a more global view of mankind and its ills was being developed. The psychiatrist was seen as a social change agent, a consultant to the agencies or governments that formulated public policies. The whole world became psychiatry's catchment area, and for such visionaries psychiatry itself became more a partner of sociology and political philosophy and less a sister of the other branches of medicine.

Even as this new 'global' – perhaps even 'intergalactic' – psychiatry was devising new ways to examine the world, it focused its analytic eye on its own functioning. Psychiatry came under the same reappraisal that society was undergoing, and new insights cast doubt on some of the old myths that had come to be accepted as basic truths. Psychiatry had held the foolish notion that the mental health reformers of the 1840s had rescued the mentally ill, that they had saved people unable to defend themselves against the ravages of a predatory, heartless, rapacious, exploitative, self-centred society by building havens for them in asylums and retreats. Thus in the United States the state mental hospital system had been born. But in the twentieth century, this was interpreted as having snatched the person from the loving arms of his family and community, depriving him of the benefits society has devised for its members (muggings, murders, release from back wards to be knifed in back alleys), imposing on him a new illness, the social breakdown syndrome, and using it as an excuse for invading his privacy, assaulting his body, and blunting his mind with treatments that did more harm than good.

The third psychiatric revolution

So another wave of reform engulfed us in the 1960s as nationwide programs were mounted to get patients out of state hospitals and place them into the community. The community mental health movement was touted as the third psychiatric revolution; one of its major elements was the move from a medical model to a systems/economic/political power model. Hospitals were to be eliminated in accord with economic policy decisions. Meeting the real needs of patients would highlight the repressive, social control aspects of the medical model, the discriminatory and segregative organization of mental institutions and of academic psychiatry. We marched under the banners of deinstitutionalization, normalization and mainstreaming in our drive to get patients back to their communities. We did succeed in getting some back, of course, but their expulsion from mental hospitals was no guarantee that they had disappeared or that their illness had been eradicated.

As Mencken observed, for every human problem there is a solution that is simple, neat – and wrong. At the present time, the patient is seen as being treated best within the setting that is presumed to have induced or contributed to his illness. For more than two decades, it has been the official policy in both the United Kingdom and the United States to develop alternatives to hospitals in hopes of closing them. The policy seems to be based, at least in part, upon the logical fallacy that since bad hospitals are bad for some patients, any hospital is bad for any patient. The continuation of the policy ignores mounting evidence that the least restrictive alternative may not always be the most beneficial alternative, and that we are not yet able to maintain every mentally ill patient outside a hospital environment.

Furthermore, the emphasis on community care has always been linked with the idea of treatment in small psychiatric units in general hospitals. Local communities, unfortunately, have not always been eager to adopt each new idea that psychiatrists and social policy planners develop, and they have often been slow to accept responsibility for the aftercare that is an essential part of our grand plan. With the worldwide recession of the 1970s there was a cutback in funding for *all* hospitals – and, as usual, it was most severe for psychiatric units. In consequence, even the communities that are ready to adopt our policies have not been able to afford them.

This is not to deny the contributions of the community mental health movement, but only to raise questions as to how it managed to go wrong. It also raises the question of how it was possible in the first place. Technologic developments, and in particular the development of psychopharmacologic agents, certainly made it medically possible to manage patients outside institutional settings. Of equal or even greater importance, though, was the economy, for when the mentally ill were defined in the United States as disabled they became eligible for federal support. States and counties could rid themselves of responsibility for chronic patients by discharging them, at which point the federal government would have to pick up the tab. But most important of all was a third factor, the setting of vast social change within which both the foregoing occurred.

The rise of consumerism

On the heels of World War II arose a new egalitarianism, manifested in several ways. One was a questioning of political and social authority, a widespread attitude asking 'What right have you to tell me what to do?' and a rejection of old attitudes and values, as exemplified by the sexual revolution, the various 'liberation' movements, and 'disestablishmentarianism'.

Another manifestation was an assault on all class distinction, starting as an understandable and laudable attempt to pull the underprivileged and the disadvantaged up, and ending for some in a demand that all special rank, status, or privilege be torn down. 'Entitlement' is a favorite word in this connection; for some it seems to mean 'If you can't *give* me a Rolls Royce, at least you should sell it to me at Volkswagen prices.'

The postwar knowledge explosion that brought technologic advances also produced a learning explosion. People know more than they used to, even about technical and professional matters. As a result, they are no longer content to leave decisions about their lives and their welfare to others. Nowadays they ask, 'What are you going to do *to* me, for I have a right to know in every detail and to agree or disagree with what you propose.'

Of course they continue to ask, 'What can you do *for* me?', but in a slightly different way. They quickly go on to say, 'Nothing but the best will do!', especially if the bill is to be paid by a third party. And if the person himself has to pay, he wants to be very sure that he is getting the most for his money. Nowadays the government, trying to make good its promise of everlasting health, finds that it is paying a large part of the nation's medical bills, and it, too, is asking whether it is getting the most for its money. All this has led to an increasing emphasis on accountability, which the physician can readily accept in theory, but which he finds in practice difficult to distinguish from intrusion, interference, and a dangerous tendency to supplant medical judgment with legalistic procedures. Once legal advocacy became the major means for achieving the ends of mushrooming consumerism, the physician found himself facing a new world of adversaries. That, combined with the continuing knowledge and technology explosion, forced him into new ways of defining and discharging his responsibilities, into considering a new kind of ethics.

For psychiatry the consumerism movement has been particularly difficult, as technologic advances outstrip medicine's ability to predict their impact. It has highlighted a host of ethical dilemmas that all physicians face. Abortion, organ transplantation, and genetic engineering, for example, raise very difficult questions for which there are no satisfactory answers, although society presses physicians to give answers even as it readies itself to attack them for whatever decisions they reach. Because psychiatry is, in fact, different from medicine in several respects, it faces additional problems.

For one thing, even though our patients are severely dysfunctional, often from an early age, they do not die; they come to be an increasing social and economic burden on a society newly obsessed with cost consciousness.

For another, psychiatry deals with questions of guilt and conscience, soul and mind, attitudes and values, freedom to think and to act, the relationship of individual to society. Psychiatrists and other mental health workers deal with patients whose disorders are expressed, not as an inflamed appendix, but as distortions in social behavior and emotional relations. The psychiatrist must therefore deal not only with the patient's pain but also with his family's and society's attitudes and demands, including standards for employment and education, community expectations about social conformity and actions in public, and the definition of all of those in legal imperatives.

Another factor is that the psychiatrist is held responsible for the behavior of his patient, even as he is accused of irresponsible interference with that patient's freedom. Currently, one of his most obdurate and painful decisions (to borrow Sir Martin Roth's phrase) is that between his duty to preserve confidentiality and his 'duty to warn' those who might fall victim to his patient's impulses.

Finally, there is widespread fear, not too difficult to understand, that psychotechnology may be used to gain social control with mind-altering drugs, electrode implantations, psychosurgery, operant conditioning, and the like.

The welfare and therapeutic states

The welfare state, the *parens patriae* concept in action, began with aid to the poor and public education, and it continues to expand into multiple areas of living. Concurrent with that development, the criminal law system in the United States has undergone a gradual process of divestment as a result of which various classes of criminal offenders by previous standards are no longer subject to its sanctions. The sin of yore is the sickness of today.

Designating undesirable conduct or even undesirable viewpoints as illness rather than as crime has been a major earmark of this century. Thomas Szasz and Ivan Illich, among others, have commented on the dangers of such an interpretation of human problems, and I shall not repeat their strident criticisms here. One need not agree with one's critics in order to recognize the kernel of truth in their attacks.

That kernel is the knotty question of what illness or disease is, and in particular how it is to be differentiated from sin, or crime, or creativity. Much of the trouble we have in relation to those issues seems to be coming from outside psychiatry, medicine, and science, and we frequently decry the intrusions of government, civil libertarians, consumer advocates, and antiscience theorists into the practice of medicine. Yet within psychiatry itself we face contradiction and controversy, not the least of which is our disagreement about diagnosis and labeling, our insecurity in differentiating between variation and disease, in drawing the line between disease, potential disease, and being at risk for disease. We espouse the medical model and deny that we follow society's mandate in applying labels of sickness. But now that tobacco addiction has been decreed an illness, we wonder whether last year's smoker may have to enter a rehabilitation program to get this year's job.

It does seem, unfortunately, that the welfare state cannot long accept a passive role of human support for what already exists. It must eventually embark on active programs designed not only to relieve but to prevent crime, delinquency and poverty, to improve or cure the disadvantaged and the deviant. The merger of the welfare state with the reforming drive of the social and behavioral sciences has produced the therapeutic state, which presents unique problems for the psychiatrist.

The psychiatrist is often expected to deal with behavior that does not conform to a family's or a community's standards, but is not viewed as a dysfunction by the subject. Is the subject sick, or deviant, or merely 'doing his own thing'? Is it really his family's problem, for not understanding the younger generation? Or is it society's problem, for demanding the impossible and then maneuvering the psychiatrist into making its decisions?

Who makes the decisions that affect the lives of people? Who says they are qualified to decide? Once they start, when can they stop? Does accepting the challenge in the first instance mean they have taken on a responsibility only society can relieve them of, or can they turn their decision-making on and off at will? And if it is truly their choice to make, how do the rest of the people know at what level they are operating? Once given such awesome power, do they have it forever after, do they always exercise it? Who controls them, to whom are they responsible? What can they do with the information they have, and who can gain access to it?

Those who might finally receive the label of 'patient' are understandably apprehensive, since the treatment label engenders at least as much suspicion and hostility as does the criminal label. Those potential patients fear that in the name of therapy, society will impose upon them controls over their behavior that it ought to have no concern about. They suspect that the therapeutic state has tools of human control that are far more oppressive than the sanctions possessed by the criminal model.

There has been an emphasis in recent studies on risk factors, elements predisposing to the later development of disease. Although epidemiologic studies have often devoted themselves to identifying putative risk factors for various diseases, not even the scientific community has always been aware of the tentativeness of their implications. Only rarely have studies even considered the need to quantify the risk for any individual, to determine the relative importance of any one factor to the many others that are assumed to predispose to the disease in question, to determine whether the factors identified constitute all the factors predisposing to the disease in question. Finally, few studies of risk factors give more than fleeting recognition of possible anti-risk or protection factors, whose potential for offsetting risk factors might alter profoundly the likelihood of any person or subpopulation developing the disease in question.

In what has been called a second public health revolution in the United States, greater attention and resources are being devoted to preventing disease, such as programs for detecting and bringing under treatment persons with latent or undeveloped illnesses. Such programs may ultimately involve the treatment of millions of persons with drugs, perhaps for life, and often with a substantial impact on the quality of life of the treated subjects and their families (Guttmacher *et al.*, 1981).

One can broadly conceive of preventive strategies as being social, individual, or medical in nature. Social strategies try to alter social and economic practices that generate conditions injurious to health. Maintaining pure water supplies, which are free of toxic agents, and waste removal are long-established preventive health practices. More controversial are recent efforts to reduce the release of health-threatening substances into the environment and to create safe work conditions.

Prevention strategies often assume that individuals are responsible for maintaining their health, or at least for avoiding activities that endanger health. One extension of such assumptions is that those who voluntarily place themselves at greater risk for disease or injury should pay a greater share of health care costs. How this would apply to persons in dangerous occupations that guard the public welfare, such as police or firemen, has never been made very clear.

Another difficulty is that the decision to treat subjects presumed to be at risk is made under conditions of great uncertainty. Like the psychiatrist trying to differentiate between the social drinker and the alcoholic, between schizoid or schizotypal personality and schizophrenia, the internist who makes 'diagnoses' of hypertension, for example, finds there is no method of determining whose pressure will rise, whose will fall, and whose will remain in the borderline range.

Because of the nature of psychiatry, the arguments over what it might do to the lives (and reputations) of people has added to the public's distrust of it. The public, no less than psychiatrists themselves, recognize the clash between its dual functions of helping patients and of helping society to run more smoothly. Any number of issues spring to mind, one with which we are currently struggling being that very complex debate about privacy and confidentiality, involving both third-party payers and insurance claims on the one hand and research efforts on the other. Health care today is a triangle of patient, doctor, and proctor; quite clearly, the proctor will gain access to some information about the patient that heretofore only the doctor was privy to. The questions are: how much information is needed to satisfy the legitimate requests of the third party, and who will have access to it once the information has been given? It is clearly proper to resist unnecessary or illegal encroachments upon a patient's right to privacy, but it is hardly defensible to assert that there can be no encroachment.

Concerns about the role that medicine and, in particular, psychiatry might play in the growing therapeutic state have brought new reformers on the scene. They appear in two main guises. One is the antiscience theorist, who argues that since most illness is socially induced, there is at best an expensive 'window-dressing' role for medical science in the prevention or treatment of disease; that medical intervention only upsets the natural balance, which is more suitably maintained by naturopaths or other health cultists; that medicine fosters survival of the *un*fit and thereby endangers the very society it would treat; and that twentieth-century treatments harm more often than they help.

In the pro-naturalistic and antimedical bias of such a climate, the clinician may not be free to choose the treatment that he has scientific reason to believe will be the best for the patient. Such treatments as electroconvulsive therapy (ECT) are the first to fall victim, and next to fall will be 'invasive' injections, or anything that might be claimed to interfere with the subject's liberty or rights.

Not radically different from the antiscience theorists in their conclusions, and sometimes even more abrasive in their methods, is a second brand of reformer, the consumer advocates. They distrust the establishment, bureaucracy, and professionalism (which they view as the cornerstone of the health 'industry'). In psychiatry, consumerism has focused on issues of civil rights, such as the right of the patient to have a say in whether he is to be treated at all; his right to a voice in planning the treatment program; the balance between individual and social needs, between civil rights and medical needs; indications for involuntary admission and enforced treatment; the definition of informed consent; preservation of confidentiality; determination of who owns or has access to the medical record; the role of psychiatry in assessing guilt or innocence, in predicting dangerousness, in determining the presence and extent of illness.

Psychiatrists more and more find themselves in a novel and often conflicting relationship with lawyers, each professional trying in his fashion to improve the lot of his patient (or client). From one perspective, the major tenet of the civil libertarian seems to be that the psychiatrist and his clinically based opinions are not to be trusted, that the patient must be protected at every turn of the road by a lawyer, no matter how costly, cumbersome, or irrelevant his solicitous ministrations might be. The assumption is that hospitalization is always the least desirable or the most restrictive alternative, or both, even as the nation recoils in horror at the indignities committed under the banner of 'deinstitutionalization'.

It is also assumed that the treatment process must be rigidly codified and standardized. The result is to obstruct access to treatment and destroy all possibility of continuity of care. The doctor–patient relationship is transformed into an adversary process that strips the physician of all power to make clinical decisions. Non-physicians define the specifics of treatment while the medical professional has at best an adjunctive role in preparing reports for the scrutiny of the judiciary or other reviewing authorities.

In their preoccupation with the mechanics of monitoring, the civil libertarians would reduce psychiatric practice to a series of mandated steps, and by eliminating all art from medicine would convert it into a technologic arm of the law.

Treatment review mechanisms have been proposed, and one for psychotropics, for example, leaves no room for change or modification in accordance with advancing knowledge. The recommended intimate and restrictive involvement of review committees in clinical, not legal, issues raises the specter of such committees ultimately deciding, perhaps by simple majority vote, what dose may be given to any patient, at what frequency, and for what period of time. No notice is taken of the countless variations produced by patients with different complaints and disorders, different levels of awareness and insight, different degrees of knowledge and competence; by families whose wants may not coincide with the patient's, whose tolerance for abnormality is wavering and uncertain, whose resources may not be equal to the demands of the ideal treatment plan; by treatment facilities and personnel whose capacities and competencies vary.

Thucydides counseled that careful study of the past frees one from repeating earlier errors. In medicine, clinical trials provide a procedural means by which to learn from past mistakes. The 'pure' practice of medicine, however, when only one effective option exists, is rare. The specificity demonstrated by penicillin for pneumococcal pneumonia and insulin for diabetes, highly desirable though it may be, more often than not is unattainable. More typically, medicine offers less than perfect remedies, and physicians make choices based upon each patient's circumstances (Chalmers, 1982). Accordingly, securing the best fit between patient and treatment is a sensitive and delicate process. To superimpose a cumbersome, costly, extraclinical, and potentially disputatious legal tier would risk its dissolution.

The psychiatrist faces the problem of doing society's bidding by ridding it of the people it does not want (usually because it finds their behavior or, more recently, merely their ideas, unacceptable), while simultaneously being accused by that society of undue pressure or influence, of depriving the patient of his rights by putting him into the sequestered detainment that society wants.

No one would deny that psychiatry *can* be a vehicle for assault on individual rights, and it is not too difficult to understand the widespread fear of the newer technologies – mind-altering drugs, electrode implants, psychosurgery, operant conditioning, and the like. At the same time, one must sympathize with the psychiatrist pressured to control, ameliorate, or abolish nonconformity by a society that files complaints against him for doing its bidding.

Even the most ardent civil libertarian believes in a reasonable balance between the medical needs of the mentally ill and the interests of society (including both protection of society from adverse social behaviors relating to mental illness, and providing care and protection for those unable to care for themselves).

It is around the concept of reasonableness that the differences between physician and lawyer peak. By his own choice, and according to his own value system, the physician is concerned more with illness and with treatment of the sick patient than with maintenance of the public safety; for the lawyer, the opposite applies. The physician considers it desirable as well as reasonable to save the life of even one person; he finds it quite unreasonable to put a higher value on the right to privacy, for example, than on the right to life itself. The lawyer, in contrast, is likely to think in terms of all of society, or the greater number of people. The lawyer, for instance, finds the psychiatrist incapable of accurately predicting violent behavior, because data show that of a group rated too dangerous for release *only* 34.7% committed a violent crime within five years of their release. Similarly, *only* one out of every 170 people diagnosed as suffering from psychotic depression committed suicide (as compared with the US rate of one out of every 8500). No psychiatrist would claim absolute accuracy in his predictions, to be sure; but his philosophy tells him it is right and just to work on the basis of high risk figures, while the lawyer's philosophy directs him to deal only with certainties.

Some would disallow at the time of commitment psychiatric testimony about possible dangerousness to self or others (because psychiatry has not demonstrated its competence in this area), but would nonetheless require the psychiatrist to make such a prediction at the time of release. One might argue one way or the other, but hardly both ways at once.

At least in the eyes of the physician, a commitment law does not exist to provide civil rights; it exists to provide human services within limits and in recognition of the fundamental human right to freedom. To protect rights at the expense of necessary medical and psychiatric services will never appear reasonable to physicians; legal safeguards must certainly be maintained for the protection of the patient, but they should not interfere with good, prompt, psychiatric treatment. The emphasis, in other words, should be on the protection of the patient who has been committed and not on the process of commitment itself.

The differences between physicians and lawyers about hospitalizing and treating reflect the same sort of difference in basic philosophy. The physician feels his responsibility is to treat people who need treatment, even though their illnesses might make some of them say they would rather not be treated. The physician, in other words, prefers to err in the direction of giving treatment that may not be necessary, while the lawyer would err in the direction of not giving treatment even though it might be desirable or necessary. Which side society is to take must be a public policy decision. Certainly if social policy is to dictate what persons may be treated, social policy and not the psychiatrist must decide on when a person is entitled to kill himself.

In short, there are differences between physicians and lawyers, but this is not to deny the need for continuing assessment of our professional attitudes and philosophy. One must question whether the physician's determination to do what he thinks is best for the patient can be maintained only at the cost of the patient's autonomy.

As Miller (1981) points out, the conflict between the values of patient and physician is never so troublesome as when a patient refuses lifesaving treatment. Under what conditions, if any, can medical judgment override the right to refuse treatment? Is a person's right to make his own choices absolute? Any attempt to answer those questions must consider the different aspects of autonomy: is the action or decision truly free, is it authentic, has it proceeded from effective deliberation?

Free action means, first, that the action is voluntary; that is, it does not result from coercion, duress, or undue influence. Secondly, the action must be intentional; that is, the subject intends to do or submit to what is in fact done. (A patient may, for instance, agree to take a vitamin pill. But if he is given a neuroleptic, without knowing that it is something other than a vitamin pill, his action in taking that pill is not free since he did not intend to take a neuroleptic.)

Authenticity means that the action is in accord with the person's attitudes, values, and life plan and not something that seems inexplicable because it is so unexpected or unusual an action for that person.

Effective deliberation means that the subject recognizes that he is in a situation that demands a decision, he is aware of alternatives and evaluates their consequences, and on the basis of that evaluation he makes his choice. It is obvious that effectiveness depends upon adequate knowledge so that consent is truly informed. Effective deliberation also requires a rational weighing of alternatives – but the physician must be particularly careful here not to equate rational with what the physician's view is, and non-rational with any choice that is contrary to the physician's. In this aspect, rational weighing is closely allied to authenticity, in that what may justly be deemed non-rational is what is inconsistent with other values the subject holds, or where there is evidence that the subject will not persist in his stance or maintain his judgment.

The doctor–patient relationship is to some extent coercive by its very nature. Emergency situations intensify the coercive element and therefore demand that special and conscious effort be made to respect the patient's values. All else being equal, the patient's own choices, plans, and conceptions of himself prevail over other people's ideas (including the physician's) about what is best for the patient. One tactic that is sometimes helpful is to present the patient with more than one reasonable option. Offering a range of alternatives from which *he* can choose tends to limit physician paternalism and promote patient autonomy.

The answer to current tensions between psychiatry and the law is not a stronger adversarial stand on one side or the other, so that one profession will emerge the 'victor'. We should instead continue in our attempts to bridge the gap between the different conceptualizations and philosophies of the two professions. The law rests firmly on the notion of free will; psychiatry, in contrast, is primarily deterministic. The task of both professions is to forge a new coupling, to reach a compromise that will help our patients. This cannot be done overnight, obviously, and no one could doubt that we shall face a host of thorny issues concerning the relationship between psychiatry and the law in the coming years.

Psychiatry does not train psychiatrists to deal with social phenomena, to be experts in the areas of curing poverty, ending crime, or abolishing other social blights. We need to acknowledge more clearly the boundaries of our profession. A first step is to define what we are, what we know, what we can do; and at the same time to remain very clear about what we are not, what we do not know, what we cannot do.

REFERENCES

Chalmers, T.C. (1982). Who will fund clinical trials? *The Sciences* 3, 6–8.
Curran, W.J. and Shapiro, E.D. (1982). *Law, Medicine, and Forensic Science*, 3rd edn. Little, Brown and Co., Boston.
Guttmacher, S., Teitelman, M., Chapin, G., Barbowski, G. and Schnal, P. (1981). Ethics and preventive medicine: the case of borderline hypertension. *Hastings Center Report*, 11, 12–20.
Harrison, A.J. (1983). Scientists and engineers in the world of lawyers, legislators, and regulators. *Science*, 220, 911.
Miller, B.L. (1981). Autonomy and the refusal of lifesaving treatment. *Hastings Center Report*, 11, 22–8.
Stromberg, C.D. (1983). Health law comes of age: economics and ethics in a changing industry. *Yale Law Journal*, 92, 203–17.

Recent developments in relation to mental health and the law in the Federal Republic of Germany

H. HELMCHEN

In 1975 the Parliament of the Federal Republic of Germany (FRG) issued the report of an expert committee on the situation of psychiatry in this country (Deutscher Bundestag, 1975). This was not only the first comprehensive review in Germany on the care of the mentally ill, but was at least as remarkable as a reflection of the increasing attention of the public to this problem. Both the actual situation of the mentally ill or handicapped and the attitude of society towards them were regarded as indicators of the general developmental stage of society. Main issues were the care of those who cannot help themselves and the civil rights of those same people, who were viewed by some as being discriminated against and oppressed. Sometimes this public discussion has become somewhat exaggerated, irrational and unrealistic, mainly under the influence of the so-called antipsychiatric movement. But the reverse is true as well: the general concern about civil rights has been reflected by psychiatrically relevant court decisions of judges who surely did not act independently of public opinion – a special aspect of the fact that judges administer justice in the name of the people.

Some important aspects of this debate will be illustrated here by a few examples from legislation and jurisdiction which show some developments of the last decade. They indicate that the modern ability to treat severe mental disorders and new attitudes of the public towards the mentally ill deeply influence legislation and court decisions, and also that the latter have an important influence on almost all aspects of psychiatric practice. With this in mind, it is no accident that no examples are given from forensic psychiatry, the traditional area where the psychiatrist as an expert was involved with the law. The examples chosen are: involuntary hospitalization and involuntary treatment; suicide; alcoholism; access to case records and confidentiality. Each example will be discussed in terms of the basic problem, the existing legal solutions, difficulties with them, and proposed legal solutions for the future.

Involuntary hospitalization, involuntary treatment
The problem
There is no doubt that some people behave dangerously as a result of mental illness rendering them unable to control their behaviour adequately. Hospitalization is often the most appropriate measure, especially if it is part of a necessary treatment. But sometimes in such cases hospitalization and treatment can be achieved only against the will of the person in question. The problem is to balance the protection against dangerous behaviour that hospitalization would give the person himself and the public in general, against the impairment of that person's constitutional right of self-determination (Baumann, 1966; Amelung, 1983). The same problem is posed by the person not consenting to the treatment of the mental illness underlying the dangerous behaviour.

Existing legal solutions
The traditional solution of this problem was to base all involuntary hospitalization on law. After the Second World War each federal province ('Land') of the FRG enacted a special law for involuntary commitment ('Freiheitsentzugsgesetz', 'Unterbringungsgesetz') of mentally ill persons. Not the least result of Germany's experience with National Socialism was the passing of laws to protect the constitutional rights (especially article 2 of the constitutional law ('Grundgesetz')) of the mentally ill persons concerned by differentiated procedures mainly following the criminal justice model. This meant that a judge had to hear the patient in a formal trial in which a public health physician needed to justify the hospitalization and the mentally ill person was supported by an attorney. The only criterion for hospitalization was protection against dangerousness of a mentally ill person either to others (for public safety and order, or even for public morality) or to himself. These laws, however, did not provide a legal basis for involuntary treatment of the involuntarily committed mentally ill. Except for emergency cases where there was immediate danger to life, involuntary treatment was possible only after the consent of a legal guardian. The legal guardian had to be appointed by a judge ('Vormundschaftsrichter') after application of a defined procedure.

It is also now clear that a near kin is not allowed to consent instead of the incompetent patient. But it may be helpful for the physician to ask the relative about the presumable natural will of the patient in such a situation.

During the last two decades the definition of emergency has become much narrower, with the consequence that an increasing number of applications for guardianship have been made.

Difficulties

Since the last century psychiatrists have criticized the police law concept of protecting the public against danger. The civil law concept of personal self-determination prevails exclusively over all regulations of involuntary commitment, or at least is not well balanced with the concept of care and treatment for the mentally ill in question (Reuss, 1888; Ehrhardt and Villinger, 1954; Ehrhardt, 1966). So, for example, the law of involuntary commitment of the federal province of Schleswig-Holstein, in existence until 1979, stated that the treatment of involuntarily committed patients is absolutely barred (Lorenzen, 1981).

Psychiatrists, and lawyers too, further argue against the judicial principle that deprivation of freedom through hospitalization against the will of a mentally ill person implies that he has not the will of a reasonable man since he has lost his inner freedom through illness (Zutt, 1970; Wiebe, 1981). Other lawyers, on the contrary, argue that a right of self-determination exists independently of the consciousness, will or ability of a person to use it (Franke, 1967).

Psychiatrists have maintained that the formalized legal procedure of involuntary commitment does not fit adequately the needs of the mentally ill person and may harm him. For example, a depressive person may experience the trial as a confirmation of his feelings of guilt (Ehrhardt, 1966).

Other serious and empirically based criticism has gained more public attention in recent years. An investigation of the frequency of involuntary hospitalizations in the FRG in 1978 revealed extreme differences between the federal provinces (from 0.1% to 44.8%) and even greater differences between different psychiatric hospitals of the same federal province (e.g. from 0.1% to 61.1%) (Reimer and Lorenzen, 1979). The reasons for these differences are manifold and complex. For example, some hospitals are obliged to accept involuntarily committed patients while others (e.g. almost all psychiatric university hospitals) are not. There are also considerable differences in the availability and quality of community-based professional help outside the hospital and in the quality (and therefore the public image and acceptance) of hospitals themselves. There may be variation too in the threshold for perception of dangerousness, both between regions and between individuals concerned – professionals as well as non-professionals. There is also no federal homogeneity in the definition and use of the legal terms: some terms are vague and therefore differently used, while others are differently defined (e.g. in one federal province dangerousness of a mentally ill person to himself is already assumed if the subject cannot care for himself appropriately, whereas in others the criterion is used only in the case of immediate suicidality: Göppinger and Saage, 1975).

Proposed solutions

This criticism led to new laws for involuntary commitment. Since 1969 the reformed law in the federal province of Nordrhein-Westfalen has acted as a precedent for this legislative development. Today the majority of the federal provinces have reformed their respective laws. The intention of the legislative bodies to introduce or to improve the care of involuntarily committed mentally ill persons and to balance this against the need for protection has found its expression even in the title of the new laws: their general short title is 'Law for the Mentally Ill' ('Gesetz für psychisch Kranke: Psych KG'); the complete title of the law of 1969 is: 'Law for Care and Protective Procedures in Psychic Diseases' ('Gesetz über Hilfen und Schutzmassnahmen bei psychischen Krankheiten').

As before the new laws define dangerousness as the principal justification for involuntary commitment. But the weight of different aspects of dangerousness has been defined and changed. The first supposition is now the disease-dependent dangerousness of the mentally ill person towards himself, i.e. his life or health (according to the principle of the proportion of means). Dangerousness to others is the second supposition, and that only if important rights of others are in danger. Urgent treatment is permitted even if the patient refuses it. But this admissibility of involuntary treatment is strongly restricted. Treatments presenting a considerable risk to the patient's life or health, and those which may result in irreversible changes in personality, are not allowed without consent.

Furthermore, the patient has the right to be treated and relevant professional institutions are obliged to provide appropriate treatment and care. This implies the obligation to apply all measures, especially prehospital or outpatient treatment, that may prevent involuntary hospitalization. But all these measures must be accepted voluntarily by the mentally ill person concerned. In addition, the laws in different federal provinces regulate and control all procedures in different ways; some introduce an attorney for patients ('Patientenanwalt') and regular control of the institutions by a commission.

These laws do not solve the problem of involuntary treatment, especially in cases without legally defined dangerousness. It is stated explicitly that the need for treatment of the mentally ill alone is no reason for involuntary commitment. This has become an important issue since the advent of efficacious psychiatric treatments. Therefore it is proposed to develop the existing legal rules for guardianship ('Vormundschaft', 'Pflegschaft'). Currently they provide a procedure in three stages: (*a*) application for guardianship, (*b*) finding and appointment of a guardian, (*c*) control of the guardian's decision by a judge. But this procedure is too slow and clumsy. Therefore, a future task should be to adapt it adequately to the needs of the incompetent mentally ill by differentiated and unequivocally defined legal measures according to the degree and type of incompetency (Wiebe, 1981; Mende, 1983).

Desirable homogeneity of legal terms and procedures seems easier to obtain in the field of civil and social law because such a legal reform belongs to the competence of the federal legislation, whereas the abovementioned protective laws are based on order, particularly police law, and therefore belong to the competence of the individual federal provinces. On the other hand this may be a reason for the slower reform of the civil law, especially the statutes of guardianship.

Commentary

In any case the basic problem of polarity between protection against disastrous consequences of mental illness and the constitutional right of self-determination cannot be solved completely by law. Legislative and juridical obligations may foster the provision of adequate measures for maximal preservation of constitutional and civil rights of the mentally ill as well as the provision of optimal care and therapy. However, legal perfectionism may have negative consequences by way of formalistic bureaucracy with inconvenient and complicated procedures. Furthermore, development and application of better treatments as well as a reduction of discriminatory public prejudices are at least as important. It was shown that in the federal province of Baden-Württemberg the percentage of involuntary hospitalization fell from 11.2% in 1968 to 3.4% in 1977, i.e. before the enacting of the new law in 1983 (Lorenzen, 1981). Generally, unavoidable involuntary hospitalization because of disease-dependent dangerousness is estimated to affect 5% or less of the mentally ill.

In a comprehensive epidemiological investigation of violent offences by mentally ill persons Böker and Häfner (1973) found that in general the frequency of such incidence is the same as in the normal population.

Suicide

The problem

Suicide seems to pose a special aspect of the general problem of involuntary treatment (and involuntary hospitalization as part of the treatment): the person in question tries to die and the physician tries to hinder him from doing so. Some suicidal and other people fight for the right to die by suicide as an expression of their constitutionally protected right of self-determination. And there may be rare situations in which suicide can be viewed as an expression of a rational and free decision to overcome an otherwise inescapable situation that annihilates the possibility of a true human existence. However, psychiatrists argue against such a position as follows: (a) In general the motives and background of suicidal behaviour cannot be recognized immediately; therefore an irreversible act must be hindered. (b) In most cases of suicidal behaviour the people concerned do not wish to die, at least not unequivocally; most of these parasuicides lose their suicidality after surviving their suicidal acts. (c) In the case of mental illness the people concerned do not have a free will and, therefore, they must be protected from themselves. A particular problem comes from the physician's legal position as a guarantor for his patient. This means that a physician, in practice usually a psychiatrist, is obliged to hinder any suicidal acts of the patient in his care. This obligation leads to a dilemma, the need for strict control of the suicidal patient being in conflict with modern liberal attitudes in the therapeutic settings of a psychiatric hospital.

Existing juridical solutions

Since 1751 suicide has no longer been a criminal offence in Germany. However, a decision of the Federal Supreme Court (Bundesgerichtshof: BGH) in 1954 stated that suicide is against the moral law and suicidal people have no free will (BGH, 1954; Lungershausen, 1983). Therefore suicide is an accident in which the obligation for a third party to help takes priority over the suicidal person's right of self-determination. This moral argument has not remained uncriticized. But the legal rule of Section 323c StGB remains valid that every person is obliged to help another in the case of immediate danger. And, in addition, from the legal position of a guarantor, i.e. spouse and even physician, it has been decided that it is punishable to refrain from help in a case of suicidal behaviour. The physician may be sued for negligent malpractice, and there have been several lawsuits against psychiatrists during the last decade (Möllhoff, 1981).

In 1975 the Upper Provincial Court of Frankfurt/Main (Oberlandes-gericht: OLG) decided in the case of suicide by a patient with endogenous depression that with such patients 'absolutely particular and concrete measures for their protection must be met' (OLG Frankfurt, 1975). The court declared that suicidal patients and also patients at risk (e.g. those with endogenous depression) had to be secured in or referred to closed wards or at least remain under continuous control. This decision was confirmed by the Federal Supreme Court in 1977 (BGH, 1977).

This strong demand for control was put into perspective by a decision of the Upper Provincial Court of Hamm in 1980 (OLG Hamm, 1980). This court stated in the case of suicide by a female with reactive depression that the order for observation every hour at night, which was more frequent than usual, was sufficient. The court added that special technical measures such as the removal of door-latches had not been necessary and did not suit 'the modern concept of a humane hospitaliz-ation of mentally ill persons'. It should be added that the court rejected the plaintiff's accusation that the psychiatrist should not have trusted the patient's statement of improvement because she dissimulated her suicidal tendencies.

Difficulties

In this context the German Association of Psychiatrists (Deut-sche Gesellschaft für Psychiatrie und Nervenheilkunde: DGPN) stated in 1980 that it is impossible to avoid every suicide in spite of close control in closed wards. It cannot even be excluded that some patients may react suicidally if they experience such control, which undermines the necessary trust between patient and doctor. There are several possible influences on the increasing number of suicides of patients in psychiatric hospitals. This is valid too for the hypothesis that modern liberal settings in psychiatric hospitals are a major source of increasing suicides. It does not seem fair to require the psychiatrist to give his patients more and more responsibility, and then sue him if this proves a mistake in the individual case in spite of all diligence (DGPN, 1980; Bochnik *et al.*, 1983).

Proposed solutions

Some psychiatrists hope that the Federal Supreme Court (BGH) will limit the responsibility of the physician with respect to modern psychiatric therapy, including the pressures and even duress of society on both psychiatrists and patients.

Alcoholism
The problem

In our society drinking of alcohol is socially accepted and viewed as a voluntary act of the self-determining person. On the other hand alcohol dependency is viewed as an illness process which is characterized by negative psychic, physical and social consequences of continuous and intensive drinking which shows elements of lack of will-power and compulsion. The problem is to define the border where the voluntary condition starts to become involuntary and to recognize on which side of the border the individual case lies. This definition has important consequences in both criminal and social law.

Existing juridical solutions

In 1968 the Federal Supreme Social Court (Bundessozialgericht: BSG) stated that alcohol dependency is a disease that has to be treated and that the treatment has to be paid for by the national health insurance system ('gesetzliche Krankenversicherung': KV) (BSG, 1968). Previous to that decision only the secondary diseases of alcoholism had to be paid for. Since then the dependency itself as a disease has to be compensated: (*a*) if the symptoms loss of control, inability to stop and craving are present, i.e. the process of dependency has reached its critical stage as Jellinek defined it, and (*b*) if the dependency cannot be cured, improved or at least protected against worsening without medical help. However, four years later, in 1972, another Federal Supreme Court, the Federal Supreme Labour Court (Bundesarbeitsgericht: BAG), made a decision from another point of view. This court said that alcoholism is a self-inflicted illness and the onset is just the beginning of drinking (BAG, 1972). The consequence of this decision was that alcoholics do not have the same legal protection against being given notice from a job as do other ill people. Other Supreme Courts such as the Federal Supreme Administration Court (Bundesverwaltungsgericht: BVG) and the Federal Supreme Disciplinary Court (Bundesdisziplinargericht: BDG) did not uphold this decision.

In 1981 the Federal Supreme Court decided a special problem: a case in which a female alcoholic sued her separated husband for alimony. The court rejected this demand because the alcoholic was viewed as having brought about her neediness wilfully. These terms were specified as 'alimony-related wantonness' in the sense that the alcoholic recognizes the alimony-related relevance of her behaviour and overrides irresponsibly and inconsiderately the recognized consequences of this behaviour (BGH, 1981).

Difficulties

In practice it remains difficult to recognize the actual degree of impairment of the individual alcoholic's freedom of choice. Therefore decisions may not be free from bias by the expert's or judge's basic standpoint: to be inclined more to the modern 'liberal' position of personal autonomy, self-determination and responsibility or more to the 'medical' position of viewing dependency as a disease which exculpates the impaired individual and protects him against some social demands.

Access to case records and confidentiality
The problem

The physician documents findings, anamnesis and all other relevant data of his patient in the case record. He needs this record as an aid for his memory for diagnosis and treatment. However, recorded data are also of interest to or sometimes needed by agents of insurance companies, courts or other authorities, as well as by researchers. And last but not least, patients increasingly demand access to 'their' records. (The case record does not in fact belong to the patient but documents the data on his case.) Such demands interfere with the physician's legal and professional obligation for the closely guarded value of confidentiality. This is true especially for the psychiatrist, who deals with a multitude of different and highly personal data. Therefore, the general problem is to balance the patient's right to – or the physician's obligation of – confidentiality and the obligation of social welfare to examine through its agencies some of the patient's data in order to secure other rights he may have (e.g. his claim to compensation for disease-related handicaps).

A more special aspect is related to research. For some research questions, e.g. epidemiological ones, the processing of person-related data is necessary. The results of such research serve as a rational basis for improving the care of the individual patient. The problem here is to balance the patient's right of confidentiality and his right to receive the best care possible, against the physician's obligation to contribute to a scientific study designed to improve care.

Yet another aspect of the same problem is to balance the patient's right to be informed and the right of confidentiality of others. Information, and the related access of the patient to 'his' case record, serve the patient's constitutional right of self-determination. However, this access may violate the rights of third parties who have given confidential information or about whom the record contains relevant data. Another problem in this context is to balance the patient's constitutional right of self-determination and the physician's hippocratic obligation to cure the patient, since the information may harm the patient. Therefore, the question must be answered whether the will or the weal of the patient has priority.

Existing juridical solutions

Social administration

In 1978 the Federal Supreme Court stated that a case record in due order is not only an aid for the physician's memory at his will, but also a component of the careful treatment he owes the patient (BGH, 1978).

The existing contracts between health insurance in the FRG ('Krankenkasse') and the institutions of medical care, i.e. physicians or hospitals, are based on the national health insurance law (Reichsversicherungsordnung: RVO). The contracts state that the payment of the insurance is dependent on the diagnoses, about which the physician has to inform the insurance, and without the immediate consent of the patient.

Research

In 1982 the Data Protection Authority of the federal province of Baden-Württemberg stopped the only psychiatric case register in the FRG – the local case register of the Central Institute for Mental Health in Mannheim – which is the only research centre for psychiatric epidemiology in the FRG. Although no case of misuse could be found, the register was stopped because the data protection law of Baden-Württemberg states – as do in a similar way the respective laws of the other federal provinces – that it is not permissible to store person-related data indefinitely for research projects not yet defined. The Data Protection Authority also demanded written informed consent from patients for storage and use of their data for research. Further problems arise from the different (theoretical and practical) definitions of anonymity for case-related data and the degree of anonymity necessary to protect records against misuse.

As a departure from this the Federal Social Law Book X (Sozialgesetzbuch X: SGB X) interestingly declares the disclosure of person-related social data as admissible if this is necessary (1) for scientific research in the field of social services, and (2) for planning in that field by an authority, provided the protectable interests of the persons concerned are not impaired and the public interest outweighs considerably the individual's interest in confidentiality (SGB X, section 75). This federal law was enacted in 1980 and regulates all administrative procedures of all social authorities.

Access to case records

In 1982 the Federal Supreme Court published two decisions concerning, for the first time, the access of patients to 'their' case records. These decisions complement each other.

In the case of a surgical patient the decision was as follows: 'in principle the patient can claim access to the case record concerning him insofar as it concerns recordings of objective physical findings and reports of treatments (medication, operation, etc.)' (BGH, 1982a).

In the other case, of a psychiatric patient, the decision was as follows: 'Even after termination of psychiatric treatment there is no obligation in principle to give access to the case record even to a patient without symptoms' (BGH, 1982b).

The extensive reasoning of both decisions makes it clear that their practical consequences are very similar to each other. The court has accepted in principle the access of the patient to 'his' record, because 'the right of self-determination and personal dignity forbid keeping the patient under treatment in the role of a mere object'. However, in both cases access is restricted to 'objective' parts of the case record, and it is left to the physician's discretion to withhold from the patient parts of the individual case record which reflect the personal aspects of the relationship between the physician and the patient or third parties (subjective impressions, personal judgments, preliminary diagnosis, reports of or on third parties, etc.). Because these latter parts are in general much more extensive in psychiatric case records than in those of other medical disciplines, it was viewed mainly as a matter of practicability to give access in principle to medical case records while withholding those data of a personal nature and, vice versa, not to give access in principle to psychiatric case records but to allow the patient to see records of 'objective findings' and reports.

Difficulties

In 1983 the German Association of Psychiatrists (DGPN) made a statement on these fairly well balanced court decisions. It deals particularly with the so-called therapeutic privilege, because the court decisions confirm previous decisions on the patient's right to injure himself by receiving medical information. The DGPN statement outlines that such obligation of the physician possibly to harm his patient by giving him certain information is contrary to the physician's traditional hippocratic principles. Thus, jurisdiction will have some impact on the physician's view of his duty. The balance between the patient's right of self-determination and the physician's obligation to cure lies somewhere between the acknowledgement of the special quality of the doctor–patient relationship and the reduction of this relationship to that of a civil contract between two equal partners. This may unwittingly foster tendencies of 'defensive medicine'. On the other hand it may force the physician and especially the psychiatrist to think twice about his proposed treatment for the patient and to choose carefully the sometimes narrow and difficult path between overprotection and *laissez-faire* (DGPN, 1983).

Future development

The DGPN statement continues that in any case the necessary freedom of decision that is given to the physician by the above-mentioned court decisions can be preserved only by the continuing responsible and humane conduct of psychiatrists.

Summary and conclusions

In the FRG the last decade has brought manifold changes in the law and court decisions which significantly influence psychiatric practice. Their basic tendency is to protect the constitutional rights of the mentally ill as well as those of others, and to improve the care of the mentally ill. A major problem has been to balance the means that aim to realize these sometimes contradictory objectives.

It seems desirable to monitor objectively the consequences of these recent and fairly rapid developments in the law. Furthermore, there is a need for both conceptual and empirical research, at least in special fields such as suicide in psychiatric hospitals or the informed consent of mentally ill persons (Helmchen and Müller-Oerlinghausen, 1975, 1978; Helmchen, 1981, 1982).

The author's thanks for help in translation are due to Mrs Jane Helmchen, MA.

REFERENCES

Amelung, K. (1983). Die Einwilligung des Unfreien. *Zeitschrift für die gesamte Strafrechtswissenschaft*, 95, 1–31.
BAG (1972). Urteil vom 07.12.1972, AZ 5 AZR 350/72. *Neue Juristische Wochenschrift*, 26.2, 1430–1.
Baumann, J. (1966). *Unterbringungsrecht*. Mohr, Tübingen.
BGH (1954). Urteil vom 10.03.1954, AZ 6 SSt 4/53.
BGH (1977). Urteil vom 06.12.1977, AZ VI ZR 170/75.

BGH (1978). Urteil vom 27.06.1978, AZ VI ZR 183/76. *Neue Juristische Wochenschrift*, 31.2, 2337–9.
BGH (1981). Urteil vom 08.07.1981, AZ IVb ZR 593/80. *Neue Juristische Wochenschrift*, 34.2, 2805–8.
BGH (1982a). Urteil vom 23.11.1982, AZ VI ZR 222/79. *Spektrum der Psychiatrie und Nervenheilkunde*, 12, 39–49.
BGH (1982b). Urteil vom 23.11.1982, AZ VI ZR 177/81. *Spektrum der Psychiatrie und Nervenheilkunde*, 12, 50–6.
Bochnik, H.J., Böker, F., Böhme, K., Dörner, K., Köster, H., Maier, S., Lungershausen, E., Pohlmeier, H., Ritzel, G. and Wanke, K. (1984). Thesen zum Problem von Suiziden während klinisch-psychiatrischer Therapie. *Neue Zeitschrift für Strafrecht*, 4, 108–9.
Böker, W. and Häfner, H. (1973). *Gewalttaten Geistesgestörter*. Springer, Berlin, Heidelberg and New York.
BSG (1968). Urteil vom 18.06.1968, AZ 3 RK 63/66. *Breithaupt: Sammlung von Entscheidungen*, 57, 809–11.
Deutscher Bundestag (1975). *Bericht über die Lage der Psychiatrie in der Bundesrepublik Deutschland: Zur psychiatrischen und psychotherapeutisch/psychosomatischen Versorgung der Bevölkerung.* Drucksache 7/4200.
DGPN (1980). Stellungnahme zum 'Suicid-Urteil' des OLG-Frankfurt vom 05.05.1975 (AZ: 1 U 136/74) bestätigt durch Beschluss des BGH vom 06.12.1977 (AZ: VI ZR 170/175), *Nervenarzt*, 51, 573.
DGPN (1983). Einsicht des Patienten in Krankenunterlagen. Stellungnahme der DGPN. *Spektrum der Psychiatrie und Nervenheilkunde*, 12, 56–60.
Ehrhardt, H.E. (1966). Die Unterbringung des psychisch Kranken als ärztlich-rechtliches Grenzproblem. Zur Kritik der Unterbringungsgesetze der Bundesländer. *Nervenarzt*, 37, 107–10.
Ehrhardt, H.E. and Villinger, W. (1954). Rechtssicherheit und Gesundheitsschutz bei psychisch Kranken. *Nervenarzt*, 25, 37–42.
Franke, W. (1967). Die Zwangsunterbringung unberechenbar potentiell gefährlicher Geisteskranker durch die öffentliche Gewalt. *Neue Juristische Wochenschrift*, 20.1, 281–3.
Göppinger, H. and Saage, E. (1975). *Freiheitsentziehung und Unterbringung*. Beck, Munich.
Helmchen, H. (1981). Aufklärung und Einwilligung bei psychisch Kranken. In *Psychiatrie und Rechtsstaat*, ed. M. Bergener, pp. 79–96. Luchterhand, Neuwied-Darmstadt.
Helmchen, H. (1982). Ethical and practical problems in therapeutic research in psychiatry. *Comprehensive Psychiatry*, 23, 505–15.
Helmchen, H. and Müller-Oerlinghausen, B. (1975). The inherent paradox of clinical trials in psychiatry. *Journal of Medical Ethics*, 1, 168—73.
Helmchen, H. & Müller-Oerlinghausen, B. (1978). *Psychiatrische Therapie-Forschung. Ethische und juristische Probleme*. Springer, Berlin, Heidelberg and New York.
Lorenzen, D. (1981). Zur Problematik der Unterbringung psychisch Kranker in psychiatrischen Krankenhäusern. In *Psychiatrie und Rechtsstaat*, ed. M. Bergener, pp. 130–50. Luchterhand, Neuwied-Darmstadt.
Lungershausen, E. (1983). Ethische und juristische Aspekte von Suizidhandlungen. In press.
Mende, W. (1983). Psychiatrische Implikationen zur Vorbereitung einer Neuordnung des Rechts der Entmündigung, der Vormundschaft und

Pflegschaft für geistig Behinderte sowie der Unterbringung nach Bürgerlichem Recht. Expertise für den Bundesminister der Justiz, Bonn.

Möllhoff, G. (1981). Suicid im Krankenhaus. In *Psychiatrie und Rechtsstaat*, ed. M. Bergener, pp. 97–115. Luchterhand, Neuwied-Darmstadt.

OLG Frankfurt/Main (1975). Urteil vom 05.05.1975, AZ 1 U 136/74.

OLG Hamm (1980). Urteil vom 26.11.1980, AZ 3 U 84/88.

Reimer, F. and Lorenzen, D. (1979). *Verzeichnis von Behandlungseinrichtungen für psychisch Kranke. Bundesrepublik Deutschland und Berlin (West)*. Enke, Stuttgart.

Reuss, H. (1888). *Der Rechtsschutz der Geisteskranken auf Grundlage der Irrengesetzgebung in Europa und Nord-Amerika*. Rossberg'sche Hof-Buchhandlung, Leipzig.

Wiebe, A. (1981). Familienrechtliche Unterbringung – eine Alternative zu den Psychisch-Kranken-Hilfegesetzen. In *Psychiatrie und Rechtsstaat*, ed. M. Bergener, pp. 116–29. Luchterhand, Neuwied-Darmstadt.

Zutt, J. (1970). *Freiheitsverlust und Freiheitsentziehung*. Springer, Heidelberg, Berlin and New York.

Psychopathy and dangerousness

WILLIAM H. REID

There is an old salesmen's and actors' axiom which goes something like this: If one's intended audience can be convinced of the premise upon which some subsequent argument will be based, then 'selling' the final product – be it an automobile or a dramatic portrayal – is easy. The title chosen for this paper might convey a premise of virtual equivalence between the two terms 'psychopathy' and 'dangerousness'. I do not entirely accept that premise, and hope that by the end of this paper the concept of psychopathy as I have come to know it will be elucidated and that of dangerousness broadened.

Psychopathy

First, the business of elucidation. I will not pretend to define 'psychopath' here. I would draw attention, however, to the probable differences between different psychiatrists' definitions of the term, and differences between possible intellectual, impressionistic, and practical ways of viewing the disorder and its victims. There are intellectual, or at least administrative, differences between the meanings of the term in Great Britain and the United States. One can see these by perusing the work of many psychiatrists, including Craft, Cleckley, Jenkins, and others (Jenkins, 1960, 1973; Craft, 1965; Cleckley, 1976). The mental image or impression which is conjured up by the term 'psychopath' is of course a personal one. In my own case I must admit that it is based in large part upon conversations at my father's knee. He is a psychiatrist, not a psychopath.

Finally, after all of the scholarly and artful discussion is done, one must from time to time deal with real people. Some are individuals who are ruining their own lives; some are family members confused and saddened by their offspring, and some are the perpetrators or victims of violent acts.

The above notwithstanding, this paper is written with a clinical bias toward a 'disease' model of psychopathy or antisocial personality. It is a mistake to describe psychopathy solely on the basis of outward manifestations. All human behavior represents series of final common pathways of tremendously complex internal and external events. Dangerousness or criminality is no more pathognomonic of psychopathy than abdominal tenderness is of appendicitis. There is no outward trait or simple pattern of behaviors which is sufficient to establish the diagnosis.

One thus separates the adjectives 'antisocial' and 'psychopathic' from the nouns 'psychopath' and 'psychopathy', and from the phrase 'antisocial personality'. This may seem old hat; however, misunderstandings of definitions persist in the minds of professionals and lay-persons alike. It is as though someone were trying to give psychopaths a bad name.

Case examples

I have recently been involved in several murder trials in which the defendants – who clearly had committed the act of killing – had siblings of similar genetic make-up and developmental environment (in one case an identical twin). Careful evaluation of the siblings raised a number of academic and philosophical questions, many of which were not germane to the legal issues at hand.

Case number one

In one situation clearly related to characteristics of antisocial personality, two brothers went through childhood, adolescence and early adulthood fulfilling every American '*DSM-III*' criterion for antisocial personality (*DSM-III*, 1980). Their criminal careers were intertwined, although neither expressed a particular liking for the other, preferring to describe their closeness as a situation in which they were necessarily 'together against the world'.

At around age thirty, one brother, 'Johnny', apparently moved away from criminality as a way of life (although he retained many other psychopathic characteristics). The other, 'Tom', continued the cycle of robberies, burglaries, arrests, and convictions. The brothers' descriptions of themselves and each other agree with available records that up to this time neither had apparently routinely engaged in violence (although Johnny had a history suggestive of poor impulse control and sadism), nor had either committed heinous crimes such as murder or rape (excluding statutory rape).

At age thirty-three, Johnny was arrested. It became apparent that since stopping property offenses he had engaged in a series of brutal seductions, rapes, and torture slayings. At about the same time, Tom, then thirty-five, completed several years of psychotherapy with an excellent prison psychologist, was released, and began a slow reintegration into society.

At present, some three years later, Tom is still 'straight' and, in my opinion, is well on the way to successful rehabilitation. When asked whether he sees differences between himself and Johnny, his answer is thoughtful and clear: when they were criminals 'together against the world', they were very much alike, except that Johnny had a greater orientation toward purposely hurting others. Eight years later, when both are in their mid-to-late thirties, there are great differences. Johnny's impression, voiced independently from a jail cell, is similar.

Both brothers speak of a 'power' and of a 'dark side' not unlike a theme of the popular movie *Star Wars*. Johnny, the sadistic murderer, feels the 'power' as a sometimes helpful, sometimes destructive incarnation of his father – executed thirty years ago for several cold, sadistic murders – which has nourished and protected him since his rather chaotic childhood. Tom has a different philosophical view, feeling that Johnny somehow *allowed* his 'dark side' to permanently take him over.

Both are concerned about the fate of Johnny's son, Johnny, Jr. His father's fantasy is to write him letters just before his execution, telling him of the power which is within him, teaching of its advantages, and warning him of its dangers.

Incidentally, the 'dark side' metaphor, complete with its potential for prophecy to future generations, is a striking characteristic of many dangerous psychopathic individuals. Similar terms are used by other members of their families, their defense attorneys, and even their psychotherapists. Whether the concept represents a denial-related mode of thinking which alleviates some of the anxiety and confusion within both the psychopath himself and those around him regarding the psychopath's behavior – a convenient metaphor for discussion and description – or merely an attractive, and sensational, way of packaging one's frightful attributes, is unclear to me.

Case number two

Mr Jones has a classic history of truancy and delinquency in childhood; many brief marriages; dishonesty and criminality as an adult; and the coldly planned seduction, torture, and murder of at least ten individuals. A forensic psychiatrist of my acquaintance had no difficulty making a primary diagnosis of antisocial personality, based upon the *DSM-III* criteria. A second psychiatrist, more experienced in the study of particular patterns of murder, suggested that a more appropriate

primary diagnosis was that of classic sexual sadism, *DSM-III* notwithstanding. My own interviews with the defendant and others, and record
review, indicated, to my own satisfaction, the presence of a severe
developmental disorder which might be called 'neurotic' because of
strong overtones of both Oedipus and family prophecy. In particular, the
central emptiness described in true psychopathy by Karpman (1941) (as
'anethopathic') and later by the author (Reid, 1978c) was not present.

Tom and Johnny, who are not particularly unusual within this already-
unusual study group, both filled *DSM-III* criteria for antisocial personality (and almost filled criteria for borderline personality). This fact
illustrates an important part of my view of the true psychopath. Was one
misdiagnosed, as illustrated by his life change? Or were both truly
psychopaths, one of whom (for whatever reasons) was able to change,
perhaps in response to treatment? To take either position, one must re-
examine at least one view commonly held with respect to psychopathy:
either that present diagnostic criteria are sufficient to define these
persons, or that antisocial personality is a virtually untreatable condition.
In my opinion, both of these premises are, at the least, incomplete.
Expansions of this opinion, and supporting data, are available elsewhere
in the literature (Carney, 1978; Reid, 1978a, b, 1981a, b; Marohn et al.,
1980).

Mr Jones exhibited an interesting group of characteristics which might,
on the one hand, differentiate him from the true psychopath but on the
other support a view of organic central nervous system deficit as
contributory to the history and behavior of those with antisocial
personality. He showed a persistence into adult life of infantile characteristics which were often unbridled by mature, inhibiting defense
mechanisms. What was outwardly manifested as adult rage was in fact
action taken on *infantile* impulses – a two-year-old's emotions in an adult
male body, abetted by the presence of secondary process thinking.

The Jungian concept of erotic disability, as illustrated by John Edward
Talley's discussion of persistence of the *puer* into the psychopath's adult
emotional framework (Talley, 1978) and Guggenbühl-Craig's monograph *Eros on Crutches* (Guggenbühl-Craig, 1980), fits nicely into such a
hypothesis.

In the past several years there have been a few opportunities to examine
carefully the neurological characteristics of severely antisocial, but
otherwise apparently normal, individuals. Several decades ago attempts
were made to find gross electroencephalographic changes, with or
without some sort of activation technique (Rodin, 1973; Elliott, 1978). As

these did not prove fruitful, neurophysiologists explored more reliable, although still very subtle changes in centrally related peripheral neural function (Hare, 1970, 1975). Hare, Mednick, and others have made important psychophysiologic inroads into not only some descriptors of antisocial personality but potential causes as well. For example, the recovery limbs of certain physiologic conditioning curves have some characteristics which might, in theory, be used to predict a deficiency in the psychopath's ability to 'learn from experience' (Hare and Schalling, 1978; Mednick & Hutchings, 1978; Reid, 1978*b*).

Even more exciting, for its practical value, is recent work in the field of neuropsychological testing. I have been impressed that both the Luria–Nebraska (with which I am most familiar) and the Halsted–Reitan Batteries can provide information about intracranial abnormalities unavailable on any other clinical measure. Although usually non-specific, these are nearing a state of the art where clinical predictions of gross behavior may be possible (Golden *et al.*, 1982; Graber et al., 1982).

Dangerousness

It is not the intent of this paper to convey any lack of dangerousness on the part of psychopaths (particularly as a group). Rather, I should like to examine more closely the level of their dangerousness to individuals and society, and to proffer the thought that, from at least one perspective, these people are less dangerous than commonly supposed. In some other ways, however, they are considerably more dangerous than frequently considered.

One can differentiate predation, sadism, and irresponsibility, and stress the non-specific nature of all three of these sources of potential dangerousness. In particular, predation and sadism are not, in my view, strikingly associated with psychopathy *per se*. The person with antisocial personality is one who lives his life, often in a search for stimulation, without caring about those who may be injured. I believe that while the end result of his behavior may be a countryside laid waste with victims, unpaid bills, or damaged lives, the *absence of vicious intent* – with its psychodynamically interesting corollary, absence of any logical reason for guilt or anxiety – is consistent with a diagnosis of psychopathy. The true psychopath, then, should be separated from the predatory, crazed, or neurotically driven criminal, and is generally less dangerous than any of these with regard to specific intent to cause physical harm.

It goes without saying that victims are still victims, no matter what the intent. The pain of injuries suffered is similar whether inflicted by design, negligence, or accident. The comments which follow do not attempt to make any statement with regard to perpetrators' behavior *vis à vis* intent (a criminal matter), negligence (generally a civil matter), or true accident.

Let us now consider broadening the concept of dangerousness. At the same time, in order to free our discussion from constraints related to the rarity of the true antisocial personality, we should expand our view of the perpetrators of psychopathic – note the adjectival usage – violence to include those whose intent can readily be inferred, while excluding those whose behavior is either clinically psychotic (cf. the famous Daniel M'Naghten) or arguably altruistic (such as persons in situations for which there is a social constituency, including actions of war or political terrorism). The group which remains is broad indeed.

Here the 'victim' changes; the greater injuries now are social limitation, inconvenience, or fear itself rather than simple physical intrusion. The victim may be a community, a demographic subgroup, or an entire society. In a sense, the victim is our freedom, and perhaps even our civilization.

We have stepped out of the realm of the individual criminal and are now speaking either of violence on a social scale (e.g. riot or non-political terrorism) or of socially significant accumulations of individual events (e.g. 'crime waves'). In both cases, we are blessed with a painfully effective system of communications media which tells us what is happening across town or around the world and which, during 'up-close' feature stories, promotes our identification with both perpetrator and victim.

There are varying views with respect to the influence the media have upon potential criminals or terrorists (Miller, 1982). Suffice it to say here that to my knowledge no study has ever demonstrated a clear relationship between the press *per se* (free or restricted) and patterns of major crime or terrorism.

Identification with the perpetrator has been discussed at length in the literature; identification with the victims of faraway criminal or terrorist incidents is discussed less often. It is, however, absolutely basic to the ability of the terrorist to extort things from us: 'Kill one, scare ten thousand.' Indeed, this identification with other victims and the fear that it engenders make it possible for us to coin the phrase 'social problem'. Our identification to the point of empathy gives rise to healthy concern for our safety *and for the feelings and safety of others whom we perceive to be like us*. This marks an important difference between ourselves and the psychopathic perpetrators.

The above smacks of a somewhat disturbing dichotomy between 'us' and 'them'. As any good liberal or social anthropologist will attest, such are the seeds of prejudice and bigotry. We have no predictive psychiatric criteria for the dangerousness of others which are sufficiently effective in real social settings to allow prudent preventive measures to be taken against individuals or groups.

Professor John Monahan received the 1982 Guttmacher Award of the American Psychiatric Association for his monograph *The Clinical Prediction of Violent Behavior* (Monahan, 1981). In it, he notes the serious questions which have been raised about the absence of any evidence that mental health professionals have special expertise in making reliable or accurate predictions concerning violent or other behaviors. Predicting events that have very low rates of occurrence is, even for repeatedly violent individuals, extremely difficult. A number of studies cited by Monahan and others note the statistical ability to separate large groups of dangerous and non-dangerous persons; however, the incidence of false positive and false negative results makes individual prediction impossible in most cases (Kozol, Boucher and Garofalo, 1972; Monahan, 1973; Steadman, 1977).

There are situations in which violent behavior can be predicted with sufficient accuracy to warrant institutional control (e.g. to justify segregating a patient within a psychiatric unit). The criteria necessary for this level of accuracy (which is still not perfect) include knowledge of very recent violence, prediction for only the very near future, and the assumption that the individual in question will remain in his present environment. The last point, of course, mitigates against the advisability of predictions as to whether a patient will be dangerous after leaving the hospital, or whether an inmate will be dangerous after leaving the prison.

An argument against mental health professionals being in a decision-making role with respect to the incarceration (imprisonment or hospital-ization) of potentially 'dangerous' individuals flows from the above facts. Although the care and treatment of individual patients must remain the province of the physician – or in some instances some other helping professional – I am in general agreement with caselaw in the United States over the past decade which has tended to place responsibility for criminal commitment or release of potentially dangerous persons in the hands of judges, not psychiatrists. The social and constitutional responsibilities weigh heavily upon the judiciary; they are outside the expertise of the medical profession.

We must, then, continue to rely upon the segregation of those proved to be dangerous in the past and upon voluntary insulation of ourselves from potentially dangerous situations in the present and future. For example, we lock our doors, stay out of certain parts of town after dark, pay a premium to live in 'safe' neighborhoods, and many of us clamor for stricter controls by the police and the judiciary.

And here is one of the greatest dangers. It is the two-horned dilemma of encroachment upon our freedoms from both the perpetrators and ourselves. On the one hand, we frustratedly give up the ability to move about as we please after dark, to take that romantic walk through the woods, to send the children to play on their own. On the other, many have suggested we abridge everyone's freedom in an effort to contain the antisocial element. In doing so we may, by our own hand, become victims before we have even been victimized.

Make no mistake; the psychopathic person cares little about your laws and mine. He turns both our rights and our abridgements of them back against us. Until society is so repressive that there are few freedoms left, he continues to act as he pleases.

It is a true dilemma; I have no answer. I am deeply concerned – even frightened – that we seem to lose either way. To make matters more frustrating, it isn't our fault. We are the victims of our own love affair with fairness and democracy, of our own civilizing empathy. Indeed, perhaps this pleasant quirk of humankind, and the grand experiment of democracy and individual rights which grew from it, will turn out to be but a brief flash in the pan of social evolution.

REFERENCES

Carney, F.L. (1978). Inpatient treatment programs. In *The Psychopath: A Comprehensive Study of Antisocial Disorders and Behaviors*, ed. W.H. Reid, pp. 261–85. Brunner/Mazel, New York.

Cleckley, H.M. (1976). *The Mask of Sanity*, 5th edn. Mosby, St Louis, MO.

Craft, M. (1965). *Ten Studies into Antisocial Personality*.
Williams and Wilkins, Baltimore. *DSM-III* (1980). *Diagnostic and Statistical Manual of Mental Disorders*, 3rd edn. American Psychiatric Association/American Psychiatric Press, Washington, DC.

Elliott, F.A. (1978). Neurological aspects of antisocial behavior. In *The Psychopath: A Comprehensive Study of Antisocial Disorders and Behaviors*, ed. W.H. Reid, pp. 146–89. Brunner/Mazel, New York.

Golden, C.J., Ariel, R.N., McKay, S.E., Wilkening, G.N., Wolf, B.A. and MacInnes, W.D. (1982). The Luria–Nebraska Neuropsychological Battery: theoretical orientation and comment. *Journal of Consulting and Clinical Psychology*, 50, 291–300.

Graber, B., Hartmann, K., Coffman, J.A., Huey, C.J. and Golden, C.J. (1982). Brain damage among mentally disordered sex offenders. *Journal of Forensic Sciences*, 27, 125–34.

Guggenbühl-Craig, A. (1980). *Eros On Crutches*. Spring Publications, University of Texas, Irving.

Hare, R.D. (1970). *Psychopathy: Theory and Research*. Wiley, New York.

Hare, R.D. (1975). Psychophysiological studies of psychopathy. In *Clinical Applications of Psychophysiology*, ed. D.C. Fowles, pp. 77–105. Columbia University Press, New York.

Hare, R.D. and Schalling, D. (eds.) (1978). *Psychopathic Behavior: Approaches to Research*. Wiley, Chichester.

Jenkins, R.L. (1960). The psychopathic or antisocial personality. *Journal of Nervous and Mental Disorders*, 131, 318–34.

Jenkins, R.L. (1973). *Behavior Disorders of Childhood and Adolescence*. C.C. Thomas, Springfield, IL.

Karpman, B. (1941). On the need for separating psychopathy into two distinct types: the symptomatic and the idiopathic. *Journal of Criminal Psychopathology*, 3, 112.

Kozol, H., Boucher, R. and Garofalo, R. (1972). The diagnosis and treatment of dangerousness. *Crime and Delinquency*, 18, 371–92.

Marohn, R.C., Dalle-Molle, D., McCarter, E. and Linn, D. (1980). *Juvenile Delinquents: Psychodynamic Assessment and Hospital Treatment*. Brunner/Mazel, New York.

Mednick, S.A. and Hutchings, B. (1978). Genetic and psychophysiological factors in asocial behavior. In *Psychopathic Behavior: Approaches to Research*, ed. R.D. Hare and R. Schalling, pp. 239–54. Wiley, Chichester.

Miller, A.H. (ed.) (1982). *Terrorism: The Media and the Law*. Transnational Publishers, Dobbs Ferry, NY.

Monahan, J. (1973). Dangerous offenders: a critique of Kozol *et al. Crime and Delinquency*, 19, 418–20.

Monahan, J. (1981). *The Clinical Prediction of Violent Behavior*. Crime and Delinquency Series Monograph. US Department of Health and Human Services, Washington, DC.

Reid, W.H. (1978a). Diagnosis of antisocial syndromes. In *The Psychopath: A Comprehensive Study of Antisocial Disorders and Behaviors*, ed. W.H. Reid, pp. 3–6. Brunner/Mazel, New York.

Reid, W.H. (1978b). Genetic correlates of antisocial syndromes. In *The Psychopath: A Comprehensive Study of Antisocial Disorders and Behaviors*, ed. W.H. Reid, pp. 244–59. Brunner/Mazel, New York.

Reid, W.H. (1978c). The sadness of the psychopath. *American Journal of Psychotherapy*, 32(4), 496–509.

Reid, W.H. (ed). (1981a). *The Treatment of Antisocial Syndromes*. Van Nostrand Reinhold, New York.

Reid, W.H. (1981b). The antisocial personality and related syndromes. In *Personality Disorders: Diagnosis and Management*, 2nd edn, ed. J.R. Lion, pp. 133–62. Williams and Wilkins, Baltimore.

Rodin, E.A. (1973). Psychomotor epilepsy and aggressive behavior. *Archives of General Psychiatry*, 28, 210–13.

Steadman, H. (1977). A new look at recidivism among Patuxent inmates. *Bulletin of the American Academy of Psychiatry and the Law*, 5, 200–9.

Talley, J.E. (1978). A Jungian viewpoint. In *The Psychopath: A Comprehensive Study of Antisocial Disorders and Behaviors*, ed. W.H. Reid, pp. 118–31. Brunner/Mazel, New York.

Dangerousness in social perspective*

JEAN FLOUD

Dr Alan Stone (1982) gives a list of adverse social consequences of civil libertarian and progressive reforms in American law and psychiatry. I shall not try to deal with his critique as a whole: of his 'bill of particulars' I shall attend only to the question of protecting the public. The concept of dangerousness is the villain of his piece and I shall consider it in social perspective by offering some observations on the notion of protecting the public and on the suitability of clinical assessments of dangerousness as instruments of public policy.

There is today a tension at the heart of public policy: protecting the public indirectly from the risk of grave harm at the hands of mental patients and serious offenders, by hospitalising and imprisoning them for long periods, frequently exposes those sentenced to the risk of unnecessary detention – unnecessary, that is, for the avowed purposes of treatment or punishment. Wherever the movement to block this source of injustice has been successful, the authorities have thought it necessary to make special arrangements to identify and detain a minority believed to be dangerous. But the practice of detaining people on a presumption of dangerousness carries its own risk of infringing the rights of mental patients and serious offenders; for a high degree of uncertainty is inherent in predictive judgments of conduct, and preventive measures taken on the basis of such judgments impose on those to whom they are applied a correspondingly high risk of being detained unnecessarily. The practice therefore comes under attack from reformers, who say it should be abandoned. To those who, like Dr Stone, point to the likely cost in terms of reduced protection for the public, the reformers say that this is the price of liberty and that a free society can be expected to pay it. The public, they say, must be educated to accept the risks entailed by the recognition of the rights of the mentally ill to treatment under the least restrictive

---

* I am greatly indebted at many points in this paper to discussion with Mr Ian White, St John's College, Cambridge.

conditions, and of offenders to punishment for the instant offence strictly according to their just deserts. But how far is this feasible? Can we justifiably abandon the practice of assessing dangerousness?

There undoubtedly exists a minority of mental patients and serious offenders who represent a risk, deemed unacceptable, of grave harm to themselves or others, and become the focus of public alarm if they are not locked up. Risks are perceived as dangers when fear is present; and though we know that people can be expected to tolerate the risk of some, perhaps most, ills as part of the conditions of life, we also know that certain others, especially those inflicted gratuitously and with violence, are regarded as intolerable and generate strong emotions of fear and resentment. Relief is called for, and if it is not forthcoming individuals will take the law into their own hands, with potentially serious social consequences. Unless public fears are to be altogether disregarded, which would be morally unjustifiable as well as politically unthinkable, protection must be available in case of need.

Since public fears cannot be justly disregarded, they must be justly assessed; and if preventive measures are called for, they must be justly imposed and administered. Estimates of the risk represented by persons alleged to be dangerous are indispensable for both purposes. It seems that the short answer to the question, of whether we can justifiably dispense with assessments of dangerousness, is that we cannot; but, given the unavoidable difficulties and dilemmas to which these assessments give rise, the short answer will not suffice to close the argument.

Preventive detention in hospital or prison is intended to guard against a certain risk of grave harm; but in making use of these measures we unavoidably incur another risk – the risk of imprisoning or hospitalising an individual unnecessarily. Whatever we do, one or other of these risks will eventually be realised. Some people find no difficulty in deciding the morality of action in such circumstances. They take a straightforward utilitarian line, based on social costs, and argue that we need only compare the harm done by the crime if committed, with the harm done to the potential harm-doer by the measures taken against him. If we can say with some degree of probability that a certain person will cause some sort of grave harm, then we are justified in locking him up if the amount of harm that this would do him is less than the product of the amount of harm he would do to others, if left at liberty, and the probability that he would do it. This looks reasonable enough, until you realise that the arithmetic can lead to unreasonable conclusions: for example, there is a very low probability of any one of us doing very considerable harm. But this kind of difficulty is not crucial. The utilitarian formula can be adapted in various ways to meet this and similar difficulties in application. The objection to it is more fundamental: it is that it provides no guarantee of individual justice.

Justice depends on making logical and moral distinctions between cases which the utilitarian regards in the same light – because he takes account only of consequences, costs and benefits. To make up his mind about the justice of preventive measures he applies the sole criterion of comparative costs and advantages: it is permissible to cause a certain number of injustices for the sake of a greater or sufficiently greater advantage on the whole.

But the criterion of those who take their stand on human rights, rather than utility, is justice in individual cases: if preventive measures are permissible in certain circumstances, it is only because, in those circumstances, they are not unjust. However, those on the radical wing of the human rights movement deny that preventive detention on a presumption of dangerousness could ever pass this test. They denounce the notion of 'protecting the public' as a form of words with politically oppressive potential, and they raise fundamental objections of principle to the practice of making assessments of dangerousness. In this way they undermine the basic presumption of the justice test of the permissibility of preventive detention, which is that a decision to impose it in a particular case could be the legitimate outcome of an impartial adjudication of conflicting claims between individuals, severally and collectively.

A moral choice has to be made between two risks: the risk, if we take preventive measures, that a mental patient or serious offender may be unnecessarily deprived of his rights and his liberty; and the risk, if we take no preventive measures, that some other unspecifiable and often anonymous person or persons will suffer grave harm at his hands. The human rights movement has done well to emphasise the significance of the first risk and to point the finger at those who would overlook it: people *are* inclined to assume that if the anticipated harm is grave enough, potential victims are entitled to be protected from the risk of it even at the cost of hardship to others, regardless of whether the risk can be justly shifted. But the movement has done less than justice to the claims of members of the public to protection from the risk of gratuitous attack with its attendant fears.

Protecting the public

Critics of the legitimacy of collective claims to special protection against persons believed to be dangerous point to the powerful subjective element in the perception of dangerousness, to the sensationalism of the mass media and their power over public opinion, and to the systematically self-serving character of government policies. They rest their case on their belief in the strong antecedent likelihood that for reasons of political expediency mental patients and serious offenders will be officially declared dangerous simply because the public is persuaded that they are so and is alarmed. The philosophers among the critics invoke Professor Ronald Dworkin's concept of 'external preferences' – the preferences of persons whose particular rights and liberties are not directly threatened – for policies or measures invasive of individual rights and liberties which give expression to notions of the general welfare or 'public interest'; and his theory of rights which holds that claims to protection by measures which would invade individual rights are vitiated if they depend on such external preferences. Explicitly or implicitly, it is denied that the general welfare can be composed of the rights of individuals and consequently that there can be valid collective claims of right.[1]

A collective claim conflicts with an individual claim to protection: but is the concept of a collective claim valid? This is not the place to make the formal argument but it is worth noting that there is nothing inherently mysterious or dubious about collective claims of right: they are but logical constructions from the claims of individuals severally, as members of families or work-groups, residents of neighbourhoods, cities, regions or states. However, in the matter of preventive justice, they are often thought to be mysterious because the incidence of threatened harm is indeterminate – the eventual victims are unspecifiable; and they are thought to be dubious because the risk represented by a dangerous person is diffused over a population of potential victims and the risk to a particular individual may be quite small, even negligible, depending on the size of the population under threat. Yet any one person's claim to be protected is smaller or larger in proportion to the risk he is put under; and the fact that a large number of persons can make a claim cannot outweigh the weakening of each individual claim with the diffusion of the risk represented by the potential aggressor.

These points need closer examination. What are at issue are diverse individual claims of right: the claims of individuals deemed to be dangerous (potential aggressors) to protection against the risk of unnecessary detention; and the individual claims of their potential victims to protection against the risk of harm at their hands. The latter are the logical constituents of any collective claim to protection; but the diffuseness of the risk out of which they arise and the impossibility (not merely the impracticality) of assigning the threatened harm to specifiable individuals, are said to make them indistinguishable from the concept of the general welfare as 'external preferences', which may not be invoked to justify the invasion of individual rights and liberties entailed by detention on a presumption of dangerousness. However, the argument too readily takes for granted the logical impossibility of deconstructing the collective claims of potential victims into multiple individual claims, to yield a conception of the general welfare which does not depend on 'external preferences' and which may be weighed and balanced against the individual claims of potential aggressors.

The mere fact that the risk represented by a dangerous person is diffused over a population of potential victims, though it weakens individual claims against him by reducing the risk to which each is exposed, does not of itself rule out preventive measures. So long as the risk they collectively face is not diffused at source but is attributable to a specifiable individual, there is no reason to exclude the possibility of taking preventive measures against him.

Indeterminacy may seem to present a problem in establishing even notional individual claims. If the incidence of harm is indeterminate, this may seem to rule out the possibility of such claims; but it is not clear that it does so, since the claims are for protection against *risk* of harm and this attaches to individuals. In this respect potential aggressors and victims are in like case: we cannot specify which potential aggressor will actually attack if left at large, any more than we can specify which potential victim will actually be harmed in these circumstances. More to the point is that potential victims may be anonymous. No doubt it would be possible, in many if not most cases, to identify the individual members of a population at risk from a dangerous person, but practical considerations preclude the cumbersome procedure of formulating multiple individual claims to protection and justify a collective claim – 'collective' in the sense that it is advanced in the name of them all.

The notion of 'protecting the public' can be so construed as to bring it within the ambit of a rights-based theory of preventive justice, even without conceding the further possibility (not explored here) that some claims of right may be irreducibly collective, not individual. But there remains the problem of weighing the competing claims of members of the public and supposedly dangerous persons. The pitfalls to be avoided in this exercise can be well illustrated by reference to a recent attempt at a thorough-going application of rights theory to the problem of preventive justice (Bottoms & Brownsword, 1982).

Bottoms and Brownsword are committed rights-theorists. They acknowledge that in the matter of preventive justice potential aggressors and victims alike have their rights which must, in the jargon, be 'taken seriously': potential aggressors have the right not to be detained unnecessarily; potential victims have the right to go about their business unmolested. But they insist that preventive detention always entails wrongful violations of the rights of detainees. This would be so, they assert, even if (*per impossible*, it is necessary to add) we were able to be certain that they would actually inflict the anticipated or predicted harm. In fact, as they point out, the fallibility of predictive judgments of conduct is well-documented and the risk of unnecessary detention, to which persons detained on a presumption of dangerousness are exposed, is on average in the region of 50–60%. Nevertheless, they concede, in a situation of so-called vivid danger we may reluctantly compromise with principle and have recourse to preventive detention; but we must be sure to minimise rights violations overall. They propose a 'test' or procedural formula to ensure this outcome: take the number of the persons who would be likely to suffer rights violations if preventive measures were or, alternatively, were not imposed; make a notional calculation of the rights violations entailed by each alternative course of action, weighting the violations according to their 'depth', frequency and immediacy; discount for uncertainty those affecting potential victims; adopt the course of action indicated by the smallest overall total of rights violations.

It is notable, in the context of a rights-based theory of preventive justice, that this procedure does not purport to resolve the postulated conflict between the rights of dangerous persons and their potential victims. It does not purport to do justice to the parties by adjudicating their competing claims to protection of their respective rights. It is a device for reaching a compromise in a situation in which a just solution is presumed to be impossible. There is no acknowledgement of fault or of any other possible justification for the preventive measures being contemplated (e.g. the need for treatment, in the case of the mentally ill). The assumption is that the rights of both parties stand to be wrongfully violated: the situation is construed as a moral *impasse* in which the claims for protection are in irresolvable conflict, with the paradoxical result that the recommended compromise procedure is essentially consequentialist and aggregative. (For 'rights violations' read 'harm' and minimise the overall total, without regard to the moral and logical distinctions on which, for rights theory, justice in the imposition and administration of preventive measures depends.)

In a situation of 'vivid danger', Bottoms and Brownsword insist, we are in an inescapable moral dilemma: 'Whatever we do, release or detain, we are certain that rights will be infringed. Our task is to minimise the violations of rights'. But this cannot be so. If we were indeed certain that a dangerous person left at large would cause the anticipated harm, he would be wrong. He would have no right to pursue the act which is *certain* to violate another's rights and we would be fully justified in preventing him from doing so. Likewise, in the nearest real-life approximation to such a situation, viz. a situation of imminent danger, there is no conflict of rights to be resolved: given a situation of real and present danger the potential victim may act justifiably in self-defence, or the authorities may act for him to restrain the aggressor and forestall the imminent danger. We must assume that Bottoms and Brownsword mean the notion of 'vivid danger' to be interpreted as something less than 'real and present' danger – as characterised by some significant degree of uncertainty as to the outcome – and that it is this significant degree of uncertainty which is taken to put the parties morally on a par. Thus, they contrast the uncertainty as to the outcome for others if the supposedly dangerous person is left at large, with the certainty that if he is detained for their protection his rights will be violated 'immediately and in a fundamental way'. The wrongfulness of the rights violations in each case is taken for granted; the cases are distinguished only by the feature of uncertainty, which is held to diminish the claim to protection of potential victims but not that of potential aggressors.

This, however, will not do. Potential aggressors and potential victims, like actual aggressors and victims, are in a situation that is logically and morally asymmetrical. The victim would not harm the aggressor were it not that the aggressor would harm him; but the aggressor's inclination to harm the victim is unconditional. The aggressor is in the wrong, either actually or by virtue of the risk he presents, and this entitles us to impose preventive measures upon him. Indeed, it may be argued that justice permits us to inflict more harm on one who would cause harm, for the sake of preventing him, than would be suffered by not preventing him.[2]

If the rights violations entailed by preventive measures are justifiable in certain circumstances, we cannot assume that uncertainty attaches only to the claims of potential victims. Supposing that we have established our right to deprive a person of his liberty in certain circumstances and that, furthermore, we have as a good reason for doing so, grounds for believing that he may cause harm in the future, then the uncertainty of the outcome of a decision to detain him must bear on his claim to protection, as well as on the claims of his potential victims. If we discount the claims of potential victims, to take account of the possibility that, in detaining a potential aggressor, we may be affording them unnecessary protection, we must likewise allow, in assessing the claim of a potential aggressor, for the possibility that we may be justified in taking preventive measures against him. A rights-based theory of preventive justice calls for clear-headed even-handedness in formulating the notional claims of the contending parties.

Critics of the use of the concept of dangerousness in public policy rarely acknowledge alarm or fear for what it is: a harm in itself, not to be underestimated. It is a painful, inhibiting sensation which can grossly interfere with a person's capacity to go about his affairs. Dangers are unacceptable risks. Fear transmutes risks into dangers calling for special protection. It is aroused by sudden jolts to a sense of security grounded in established expectations, particularly by a prospect of ruthlessly self-serving or gratuitous violence in defiance of the customary social and legal constraints.

How severe a jolt makes a risk unacceptable? How great must be the disparity, say, between the risk of grave harm represented, respectively, by an allegedly dangerous person and an average member of the community in which he will reside if not detained? If the serious offence rate be allowed to provide a rough measure of the latter, and the predictive value of assessments of dangerousness a rough measure of the former, it is evident that, though these predictive values are notoriously low, rarely exceeding 50% on average, they nevertheless express a risk of grave harm which is many times larger than that expressed by any serious offence rate. To detain an individual with no more than an even chance of inflicting grave harm on another is to impose on him a heavy burden of risk of unnecessary detention. But to leave him at large is to impose on others the unusual and alarming risk of confronting someone with as much as an even chance of inflicting grave harm; which is to say, someone who is as likely as not, other things being equal, to cause him grave harm. *Prima facie*, it does not seem unreasonable to deem such a risk unacceptable.

However that may be, people have no right to protection against feelings of fear unless their feelings are justified; which is to say, explicable in terms of their object. Fear is focussed on a presumed risk of grave harm. Is the fear well-grounded? Some mental patients and serious offenders produce alarm without risk and once duly treated or punished are entitled to their freedom; others produce risk without alarm and are liable to be detained for longer than would be justified on other grounds alone. Whose judgment of the risk is to prevail? The courts, tribunals and medical and penal authorities in whose hands rest decisions as to whether or not to detain on a presumption of dangerousness, have come to rely heavily on the advice of mental health experts, more particularly of psychiatrists. But the soundness of clinical assessments of dangerousness has been vigorously challenged, above all in the United States where, since the mid-sixties, court decisions to release mental patients and serious offenders against the advice of clinicians that they should be detained as dangerous have provided numerous opportunities to put these clinical assessments to the test of experience.

Clinical assessments of dangerousness[4]

There is now widespread and profound scepticism as to the possibility of discriminating with any real degree of confidence between persons against whom protection is needed and those against whom it is not. The propriety of the practice of attempting to do so is questioned, partly on this basis and partly on the basis of more fundamental objections of ethical and political principle. I have explained elsewhere[3] that I think these fundamental objections misconceived, for the most part; but this is not the occasion for considering them and I shall confine myself to the objections advanced on clinical grounds.

It seems to me that the findings of the validation studies, which have been made possible in the United States by court decisions to release mental patients and serious offenders against professional advice, are generally misunderstood. To explain why, I am obliged to consider in some detail the nature of clinical assessments of dangerousness.

The first thing to say about these assessments is that though they issue in a prediction of some sort, they are not simple predictions but predictive judgments. I shall return to this distinction shortly; for the moment I want merely to emphasise that they are *judgments*.

As Frank Knight (1936) remarked: 'The striking feature of the judging faculty is its liability to error'; and there is an accumulation of empirical evidence pointing to a high risk of error in clinical judgments of dangerousness. I have reviewed this evidence in some detail. Here I need only say that, making full allowance for its many weaknesses, both avoidable and unavoidable, the evidence tends inescapably to the conclusion that clinicians in general have, on average, little more than an even chance of being proved right when their predictions that individual mental patients and offenders will cause grave harm if left at liberty, are put to the test. Substantial validation studies in the United States have shown that when, against their advice, their subjects have been transferred to ordinary hospitals or released into the community, not many more than 50% of them, and frequently fewer than that, have actually caused grave harm as predicted.

The art of assessing dangerousness is undoubtedly a very difficult one; but there are severe, purely statistical constraints which go far towards accounting objectively for this ambiguous success rate; and this is the second point I want to make about clinical assessments of dangerousness.

The sheer diversity of human beings and their circumstances, the infrequency with which they inflict grave harm on others outside the usual social and legal constraints, and the role of chance in determining their actions, whatever their dispositions, are the prime obstacles to successful prediction. If the clinician is not drawing his subjects from a population sufficiently homogeneous in the relevant respects for its members to have more than an even chance of causing grave harm, he cannot have more than an even chance, on average, of being right in his individual predictions, however carefully and skilfully he sets about making them. Most clinicians work within populations that are administratively defined, with a higher than average probability of doing grave harm; but their subjects are still very heterogeneous. Statisticians have had only limited success in identifying populations with more than a 50% probability of causing grave harm, even when making their selection from serious offenders with formidable records of criminal violence. In any case, the clinicians cannot win: paradoxically, the more homogeneous the population from which they draw their subjects and the higher the general or average probability of their causing grave harm, the more difficulty will the clinicians have in differentiating them individually in respect of the risk they represent; for to the extent that they have been successfully preselected, so to say, for dangerousness, individual outcomes will be determined by chance. All this is a matter of ineluctable statistical logic and it justifies a pessimistic view of the prospects of greatly improved predictive values.

Nevertheless, it does not seem to me (*pace* Dr Stone) that in acknowledging these and other less precisely determinable difficulties, whilst telling courts to make use of assessments of dangerousness, the Supreme Court was 'embracing incoherence'. I think it was simply taking a realistic view of a difficult matter.

If the chances of a right judgment of 'dangerous' seem from the evidence to be, on average, about even, it follows that it is as difficult, on average, to say who is safe as who is dangerous among the mental patients and serious offenders with whom the clinicians are dealing; and the morality of action in these circumstances cannot be decided without further discussion of what constitutes a right judgment.

The clinician makes predictive judgments, not simple predictions. That is, he is not asking the statistician's simple question: How likely is it that a man like this will cause grave harm? His is the more complex question: In what circumstances would this man now be going to cause grave harm, and what is the strength or persistence of his inclination to do so in such circumstances? And, in order to make a prediction, the clinician must ask the supplementary question: How likely is it that this man will find himself in such circumstances in the foreseeable future?

The clinician aims to arrive at a sound, and he hopes reliable, diagnosis of a disposition as the basis for a prediction of future conduct which will indicate his estimate of the strength of the disposition in foreseeable circumstances over a period of time. His predictive judgment takes the form of a reasoned diagnosis culminating in a statement along the lines: I am (more or less) certain this person is a bad risk – i.e. for the reasons adduced, I judge him (with such and such a degree of confidence) disposed to inflict grave harm on someone, and unless prevented, to be (at least as likely as not) to do so within the next x (days, weeks, months, years).

The significance for such a predictive judgment of the empirical evidence, referred to above, of the generalised risk of such judgments being wrong, is often misunderstood. It speaks, of course, to the confidence which the clinician may feel in his own estimate of the correctness of his judgment, but it says nothing to the real or objective probability attaching to the individuals of whom the judgments were made. At best the predictive values of clinical estimates of individual probabilities of harmful conduct are mistaken for actual statements of risk, i.e. for real or objective statistical probabilities; at worst statistical entities (false positive or negative predictions) are mistaken for particular, misjudged individuals.

The clinician's prediction or estimate of the risk represented by an individual is part of a composite predictive judgment; it is grounded in a diagnosis of a disposition to cause grave harm. Within the statistical constraints already mentioned, the degree of uncertainty attaching to it will depend on the soundness of the diagnosis and the clinician's knowledge and understanding of foreseeable relevant circumstances. Strictly speaking, predictive judgments cannot be validated as such. The diagnosis of disposition can be tested for reliability, by comparing the diagnoses of independent assessors, and the prediction of the outcome can be tested for validity, by putting it to the test of experience. But the two terms of the predictive judgment do not stand in any determinate relationship which answers to its rightness or validity.

Having made his diagnosis, and contemplating his prediction, the clinician will want to minimise his ignorance of foreseeable circumstances (e.g. by close cooperation with social workers and other informed persons), aiming as it were to leave everything – but as little as possible – to chance. In the hypothetical ideal case, chance alone would determine the outcome, and no matter, in that case, whether, in relation to his prediction, that outcome turned out to be a false or a true positive or negative, it could not answer in any way to the soundness of the diagnosis.

It follows that a low probability of sound diagnoses is more damaging to the credibility of a predictive judgment than a low probability of a valid prediction. Though the reliability of diagnosis of dangerousness can be much more easily tested than can the validity of predictions of gravely harmful behaviour, there appear to have been few attempts to test diagnoses, experimentally or otherwise. The first results reported by investigators responsible for the WHO Collaborative Study on Assessment of Dangerousness in Forensic and Administrative Psychiatry (Montandon and Harding, 1984) are discouraging: they 'do not support the use of "dangerousness" as a scientifically or operationally valid concept'. In any case, a very high degree of uncertainty as to individual outcomes is disturbing when long indeterminate periods of confinement in a hospital or prison are contemplated. The probability of a false positive prediction of gravely harmful behaviour states the average risk of unnecessary detention if preventive measures are taken, and though its significance for the case for taking such measures is arguably underplayed by civil libertarian critics (see pp. 83–8 above), it is at present too high for comfort or complacency.

As long as predictive judgments are made in the criminal justice and mental health systems, the moral obligation to persist with attempts to improve them is inescapable; but it is an open question as to how much scope for improvement there is, since it is impossible to estimate the extent to which clinical and statistical factors respectively are responsible for present indications of the state of the art. It would be unduly pessimistic to ignore the possibility of improved diagnostic procedures whether by means of improved theoretical insights and the encouragement of research and the utilisation by practitioners of its findings, or, simply, by more care in the selection and appointment of forensic psychiatrists.

Empirical investigations have been undertaken in the United States not only to question the competence of clinicians by demonstrating the limited validity of their assessments of dangerousness, but by study of the content of their reports to the court (Cocozza and Steadman, 1976) and by the direct study of assessment procedures in action (Pfohl, 1977) to show how the false and misleading idea is fostered that there exists a quasi-medical entity, a 'dangerous person', on which psychiatrists and associated professionals in the mental health field are expertly qualified to advise courts and penal authorities. In reporting their findings, Cocozza and Steadman have taken the opportunity of charging psychiatrists with professional hubris and bad faith, with succumbing too readily to pressure to 'play the role [of expert] to meet the expectations of society'. They are said to pose as scientists but to practise 'magic', in the sense that, although claiming special knowledge and granted expert status in law, they make assessments of dangerousness which rely on empirically untested beliefs: 'they represent an excellent example of professionals who have exceeded their areas of expertise and for whom society's confidence in their ability is empirically unjustified'. Pfohl accuses psychiatrists of 'false consciousness', arguing that they serve as agents of social control, thus conniving at the perpetuation of oppression and injustice.

This is heady stuff, but it would be an insensitive and self-righteous psychiatrist who would dismiss it out of hand. It has been argued from empirical data that the level of agreement between psychiatrists and non-psychiatrists assessing the dangerousness of subjects from their case histories is generally low, and possibly no greater than that between non-psychiatrists interpreting the same data (Montandon and Harding, 1984); and that the predictive value of clinical judgments of dangerousness is no greater, on average, than if they had been reached by tossing a coin (Ennis and Litwak, 1974). But it does not follow that psychiatrists can be dispensed with as expert witnesses when preventive detention is under consideration in particular cases.

It is true that as long ago as 1789, Bentham laid down a number of common-sense rules for measuring 'the depravity of disposition indicated by an offence' and that, for all the resources of modern psychological medicine, more art than science probably goes into a successful predictive judgment of dangerousness. Nevertheless, it would be perverse to suppose that clinicians have nothing to contribute to the assessment of dangerousness from their experience of studying and explaining mental abnormality, even in cases where a propensity to inflict grave harm on others is not clearly associated with mental illness. Anyone detained on a presumption of dangerousness without benefit of psychiatric witnesses for the prosecution as well as for the defence would nowadays have good cause to complain of injustice.

What the empirical investigations do provide is alarming evidence, from mandatory reports to the court, of slovenly diagnosis by forensic psychiatrists, and a striking correlation between their perfunctory recommendations and the decisions of the court (Cocozza and Steadman, 1976). This correlation seems to indicate slovenly adjudication ('while by law the decision was a judicial one, in reality it was made by psychiatrists'), though whether this damaging inference can safely be drawn simply from the reported absence of disagreement in 86% of the cases studied, is arguable. But the direction in which reformers should be looking is clearly indicated.

It may be, as Dr Stone says, quoting the President of the National Council on Crime and Delinquency (1973), that the identification of dangerous persons is 'the greatest unresolved problem that the criminal justice system faces'. But it is a political and administrative problem, rather than a substantive problem, since there is no substitute for predictive judgments; they are all we shall ever have to go on. If they are not made overtly with expert assistance they will be made covertly without it. Given their inherently uncertain nature, it is up to the legislature to make them explicit and to limit their scope, to put them under statutory control and hedge them about with procedural safeguards.[5]

The adjudication of the rival claims of potential victims and potential aggressors is a matter for the courts or their equivalent, assisted by expert witnesses. Psychiatrists will be unavoidably and properly prominent among the expert witnesses. Adversarial proceedings present them with special problems and their professional associations should work to clarify and publicise the scope and limitations of their contribution.

As Dr Stone demonstrates, there are unintended, unforeseen and harmful social consequences of the trend towards the judicialisation of assessments of dangerousness in the mental health system. I cannot pretend to know how these might be avoided or mitigated. The trend is probably irreversible, since it takes its impetus from the powerful contemporary revolt against utilitarian and authoritarian conceptions of justice. Psychiatrists must persuade lawyers and parliamentarians of these harmful side-effects of reform and work with them to find antidotes.[6]

NOTES

1. See Bottoms and Brownsword 'Dangerousness and Rights' in Hinton (1982).
2. See Floud and Young (1981), Chapter 3.
3. *Ibid*.
4. For reviews of the empirical evidence referred to in this section, see Floud and Young (1981) and Monahan (1981).
5. Floud and Young (1981) Part III.
6. It is gratifying to note that the work is in hand. The American Psychiatric Association has approved a Model state Law on Civil Detention of the Mentally Ill (Stromberg and Stone, 1983) which directly addresses these side-effects of reform.

REFERENCES

Bottoms, A.E. and Brownsword, R. (1982). The dangerousness debate after the Floud report. *British Journal of Criminology*, 22(3).

Cocozza, J.J. and Steadman, H. (1976). Prediction in psychiatry: an example of misplaced confidence in experts. *Social Problems*, 25(23).

Ennis, B.J. and Litwak, T.R. (1974). Psychiatry and the presumption of expertise: flipping coins in the courtroom. *California Law Review*, 62(5).

Floud, J. and Young, W. (1981). *Dangerousness and Criminal Justice*. Heinemann, London.

Hinton, J. (ed.) (1982). *Dangerousness: Problems of Assessment and Prediction*. Allen and Unwin, London.

Knight, F. (1936). *Risk, Uncertainty and Profit*.

Monahan, J. (1981). *The Clinical Prediction of Violent Behaviour*. US Department of Health and Human Services, Rockville, Md.

Pfohl, S. (1977). The psychiatric assessment of dangerousness: practical problems and political implications. In J.P. Conrad and S. Dinitz (eds.) *In Fear of Each Other*. Lexington Books, Lexington, Md.

Stone, A.A. (1982). Psychiatric abuse and legal reform: two ways to make a bad situation worse. *International Journal of Law and Psychiatry*, 5, 9–28.

Stone, A.A. and Stromberg, C.D. (1983). A model state law on civil commitment of the mentally ill. *Harvard Journal of Legislation*, 2(2).

Psychiatric explanations as excuses

NIGEL WALKER

My text comes from a text-book:

> The American system of justice is based on the theory that an individual acts with free will. *A person who is insane can no longer exercise this free choice.* (Gammage and Hemphill, *Basic Criminal Law*, 1977 edition, McGraw-Hill, New York, p. 136, my emphasis)

My theme is that this is nonsense, both in the United States and in Great Britain. Or, to be more precise, that it over-simplifies the reasons why the insanity defence excuses. To make my point clear, however, I must begin by distinguishing different sorts and purposes of explanation where human behaviour is concerned.

Explanations
Explanations of human behaviour are used in at least five ways:
1. to predict future behaviour (for example in psychiatric or political prognoses);
2. to produce future behaviour (for example in elections or psychiatric treatment);
3. to prevent future behaviour (for example in child-rearing);
4. to satisfy curiosity about past behaviour (for example in history);
5. to decide whether past or current behaviour is morally or legally excusable.

This paper is concerned only with explanations of the kind which are relevant to (5); it is not about all kinds of explanation. In particular it is concerned with the sorts which seem to be offered to criminal courts when excusing or mitigating actions. At the sentencing stage psychiatrists in court – and especially in British courts – are often expected also to testify about the treatability of defendants or make prognoses about them; but that sort of testimony is outside the scope of this paper.

During – or sometimes after – the trial itself, a psychiatric explanation may be submitted to a court in support of the argument that a person is not to blame for what he did, or at least less to blame than a person in whom a psychiatrist could not find any definite abnormality.[1] The classic situation is psychiatric evidence in support of the insanity defence. It is true that in present-day Britain this is a rarity; but it is not so rare in the United States or British Commonwealth, and may well be revised in some form, especially if the Butler Committee's proposals reach the statute-book: a possibility which is considered in Appendix 2. In any case, the situation also arises when the defence is diminished responsibility or infanticide, and arises in some instances of automatism (I say 'some' because while the defence of automatism is sometimes based on a condition diagnosed by psychiatrists or neurologists, it can also be based on a normal accident such as a sneeze).

Explaining aberrant behaviour

In order to make my points about the relevance of psychiatric evidence to these defences, I must be allowed a short statement about the explanation of what I shall call aberrant behaviour, meaning to include not only criminal behaviour but also other sorts which are usually regarded as abnormal or at least regrettable (an example being ruinous gambling).

Possibility-explanations

When, in everyday life, we ask why a person did something surprising, we are not usually demanding a scientific explanation. That is, we are not usually asking to be told why he was 'bound to' do that, or why it was highly probable that he would do that.[2] More often, all we want to understand is his reason for behaving so oddly: how he 'could possibly' make such a fool of himself, or do something so inconsistent with what we know or assume to be his principles or objectives or upbringing. What we are usually given, and usually accept as adequate, is a little narrative, which tells us how that person came to be tempted, provoked, mistaken or whatever, so that we see how it was psychologically possible for him to act so strangely. Dray, in his book on historical explanations,[3] called these 'narrative explanations', but a more exact term would be 'possibility-explanations'.

An imaginary example would be an incident in which a guest at a meal is rude to his host, in a way which not only breaches the conventions but is out of character for the guest himself. His wife asks him afterwards 'How could you do that?', and he explains that his host's last remark had been a covert reference to an old scandal in which he, the guest, had been involved. If his wife then asks 'But did you have to let yourself be provoked' he might well reply 'No, I suppose not; but I thought to myself "It can't do any harm and he needs a lesson."' His account of the incident makes good enough sense to be acceptable as an explanation, yet implies no inevitability about his rudeness, nor even a high probability. All it does is to help us to understand 'how he could': a possibility-explanation.

Probability-explanations

It is only if Smith repeatedly acts in a strange or out-of-character way that we begin to feel the need of something more than a possibility-explanation, and to ask what it is that 'makes him' do it. In such cases we are not satisfied until we are given an explanation which tells us why it would have been unlikely that he should act in any other way. I call that sort of explanation a 'probability-explanation', meaning this term to include the very rare sort of explanation which tries to show why his behaviour is inevitable.

Probability-explanations can be equated, if you like, with 'scientific' explanations. My own view, which I have argued in detail elsewhere,[4] is that this is better than defining scientific explanations in terms of natural laws, as Hempel did; but that is not an essential part of my present argument. And it is certainly not part of my argument that the distinction between possibility- and probability-explanations applies only to human or even animal behaviour. Even where inanimate things are concerned we often accept possibility-explanations. Accidents to aircraft, failures of structures such as bridges, the appearance of an iceberg in temperate waters, are often explained by narratives involving unlikely coincidences of circumstances. As Michael Scriven pointed out engineers can often explain after the event an accident which they could not be expected to predict.[5]

Nor is my distinction between these two sorts of explanation the same as the distinction between 'reasons' and 'causes'. 'Causes' can figure in both kinds of explanation, and so can reasons. A possibility-explanation of a surprising human act usually includes a reason: but it may rely solely on a physiological event, such as a muscular spasm or a sneeze. A probability-explanation of bizarre behaviour can involve either the person's reasons or a neurological abnormality. In any case, the once-fashionable view that reasons are not the sorts of things that can be causes has been undermined by a lot of telling criticism.[6]

One more point, also relevant to psychiatric explanations although more often to sociological explanations, is that it is not only the repeated aberrations of *individuals* which seem to us to call for something more than mere possibility-explanations. Sometimes it is the frequency with which *members of a category of people* act in ways which we find surprising. The behaviour of football fans is one example. Another is the frequency of vandalism in an age-group of males, or of personal violence in a whole society. When such frequencies are substantially greater than what we regard as usual, we want some sort of probability-explanation. This situation is common in sociology, but not unknown to psychiatry.

Psychiatric explanations

So consider the sorts of statement which psychiatrists offer when asked to explain an individual's law-breaking.[7] There seem to be four of these: automatism, increased probability, reasons (including mistaken beliefs) and 'irresistible impulse'.

Automatic actions

There is the sort of explanation which tells us that the subject was more or less an automaton. Epileptic seizures used to be cited as examples of this, although thorough investigators such as Professor Gunn now seem doubtful as to whether the movements of an epileptic in a genuine seizure could ever take the same form as the purposeful actions which are required for most law-breaking. Nevertheless, a seizure while one is driving a car could cause an unintentional infraction, just as could a violent sneeze, which is the nearest thing to automatism that an ordinary healthy person experiences. The gestures and grimaces of parkinsonism or Huntington's chorea are no doubt another example. In such cases psychiatrists are in effect telling us that the subject could not help what he did; and while the meaning of 'could not help' is sometimes ambiguous, in these cases it clearly means 'was highly likely (or even certain) to move in that way even if he had wanted not to'. Such an explanation is accepted by lawyers as completely exculpating the accused, unless the defendant can be blamed for allowing himself to get into the physical state or the situation: for example, by driving when he felt a fit coming on. Such cases apart, he is regarded as being as innocent as if someone else had wrenched the steering wheel.[8] What is more, we accept the psychiatrist's or neurologist's explanation even if we do not really understand the neurological mechanics, just as we take on trust an electrical engineer's explanation of the odd behaviour of a television set.

'Increased probability'

But other sorts of psychiatric explanation are not so simple. Sometimes we are merely told that the subject is schizophrenic, or manic, or in some other diagnostic category. In what sense is this an explanation? It is only an explanation if it is implied that subjects in such categories are either:

(*a*) Certain to do what they did: but this can hardly ever be the implication.

(*b*) Highly likely to do it. This is sometimes what is implied. Examples are the suicidal (and sometimes homicidal) behaviour of clinically depressed subjects and the assaults of paranoid schizophrenics, although sometimes we are offered a more satisfactory kind of explanation in such cases, which I shall discuss in a moment. 'Highly likely' is of course a vague term: in such cases psychiatrists cannot be precise about the degree of probability. Sometimes all they can be implying is that the subject is 'more likely than not' to do what he did; sometimes they imply 'very likely indeed'.

(*c*) Merely more likely to do it than a member of the population at large. (An analogy is the 'explanation' of the malfunctioning of a television set when all it tells us is that the set is a very old one, or of some discredited make.) Thus we may be asked to excuse infanticide because the woman had recently given birth and was in a distressed state (or, to use the words of the Act, 'the balance of her mind was disturbed'). Psychiatrists cannot mean that women in such a situation are highly likely to kill their babies, for most of them don't, even if the balance of their minds *is* disturbed. The most that is implied is that this is a situation in which it is more likely than usual that a woman will do this.

I call this sort of implication 'increased probability'. It is important to realise that it is not an implication that the probability is high, or even that it is more than fifty-fifty. It is even more important to realise that apart from some special kinds of disorder there is very little sound evidence for the belief that mental disorders increase the probability of law-breaking by more than a negligible degree. Some studies in the United States suggest that they do, some do not. A very careful study of intentional homicides in West Germany from 1955 to 1964 seemed to indicate that mentally disordered people contributed no more to these than was to be expected from the prevalence of mental disorders in the population,[9] but that schizophrenics did contribute disproportionately to homicides (and suicides). The problems about all such estimates are: (i) that at any given time a substantial number of severely disordered people are either inside institutions or under supervision, which must to some extent reduce their opportunities for law-breaking; (ii) that an unknown percentage of sufferers from psychiatric disorders is 'latent' in any population, having escaped psychiatric attention.

There are exceptions, however, which make it fairly safe to say that the probability of law-breaking is raised by the disorder. One is addiction to alcohol or other mood-altering drugs.[10] I do not mean simply that the abuse of a drug makes it more probable that the addict will behave violently or dishonestly or in some other way objectionably, although this often happens when too much alcohol is drunk. I mean also that the addict will make determined attempts to secure supplies of his drug, so that if this involves stealing, or forging prescriptions, there is an increased probability of his infringing the law. On the other hand, the diagnosis of addiction does not predict what specific form the law-breaking will take: only knowledge of his past conduct will do that, and by no means infallibly.

Interestingly, we do not regard such law-breaking as being excused by the addict's craving, although the causal link is both obvious and strong (that is, one which makes the dishonesty very probable). No doubt the reason is that we blame the addict for the addiction, but this is by the way.

There are also pseudo-exceptions. These are diagnoses which are more or less based on the sort of conduct for which they are offered as explanations: so much so, indeed, that they are sometimes called 'circular' explanations, for instance by Lady Wootton.[11] Thus 'aggressive psychopaths' do seem more likely than most people to commit personal violence. But since this label is little more than a description of the sort of law-breaking to which the subject is prone, to offer this diagnosis as an explanation is not really to tell us much. And the even simpler label of 'psychopath' or 'personality disorder', without some adjective such as 'aggressive', tells us even less.

What can be called for short the 'highly likely' explanation seems to be the basis for the form of insanity defence popularised in Europe by the Code Napoléon, which obliges courts to excuse the defendant if satisfied that at the time of his act or omission he was in the state called 'démence'. This is one of the revisions of the insanity defence which the Butler Committee recommended for adoption in England, together with another which I shall eventually mention (see Appendix 2).

Reasons

Sometimes, however, psychiatrists supplement their diagnoses with information which constitutes an entirely different sort of explanation. They tell us, for example, that the paranoid schizophrenic suffered from the delusion that his wife was being unfaithful, or that his neighbours were plotting to kill him, or that the clinically depressed father foresaw such a terrible future for himself and his family that it seemed kinder to kill them all.

In such cases we are not merely being given explanations in terms of weak or strong actuarial probabilities: we are being helped to understand the subject's actions. The information about his beliefs and feelings is meant to make us say to ourselves: 'I see why he did it.' More precisely, it may enable us to understand how it was psychologically possible for a person to do what he did, just as in my imaginary example of the guest who was provoked to rudeness. What it hardly ever does is to make his actions seem inevitable, or even highly probable. It is almost always possible to envisage the same person, in the same situation, deciding not to do what he did, or to postpone it.

Mistakes

Sometimes, of course, the essential part of the information is that the subject was mistaken about the nature of what he was doing. The important point about mistakes is that they usually figure in possibility-rather than in probability-explanations. I would like to be able to illustrate this from real, straightforward cases of successful M'Naghten defences. Unfortunately, as both Professor Glanville Williams and I found when independently searching for illustrative cases, these are virtually impossible to find. Those that are fully documented are those which went to appeal, and therefore are anything but clear-cut. Fitzjames Stephen gives two examples of insane mistake as to the nature and quality of one's act; but he gives no case references, and they are almost certainly imaginary.[12] Writers of text-books, however, have had to use his illustrations. One is the man who wounds someone when he thinks he is breaking a jar; the other is a man who strangled someone when he thought he was squeezing an orange. The important thing to note in both illustrations is that they merely explain to us how the man could *possibly* have done what he did. They do not present his actions as highly probable. We are not asked to believe that these individuals were in the habit of breaking every jar or squeezing every orange that they came across. All that we are being offered is a possibility-explanation.

Delusional beliefs

More often the essential part of the information is a delusional belief. Sometimes this belief is such that if true it would have been an excuse in strict law: the subject may have thought his assault necessary to ward off a lethal attack. Even if this is not so – as when, for example, a paranoid husband kills his wife's imagined lover – a delusional belief can make us understand the provocation. Very seldom, however, does it make us feel that he could not help doing what he did. We may accept that he could not help having the delusion, and yet feel that he might perhaps have acted less drastically: not every paranoid husband attacks his wife or her imagined lover. Nevertheless, we feel less censorious about his violence because we understand how he 'could possibly' have done what he did.

In practice it is almost as hard to find real illustrations of crimes committed as a result of delusions which if true would have justified them in law as it is to find real illustrations of mistakes about the 'nature and quality' of the act. M'Naghten's own delusion that he was being persecuted by the Tories did not justify his shooting the man he thought was the Prime Minister, unless – and this has never been alleged – he thought he was defending his life. I have, however, been present in court when a man was tried for stealing food from a Welsh supermarket; he thought that he had the status of a prophet of God, with the duty of reforming the Welsh, and therefore had the right to enough food to sustain him even if he could not pay for it.[13]

Mistaken moral judgments

Even more interesting is the attitude of our courts to mistakes about moral wrongness. The judges who framed the M'Naghten Rules almost certainly meant that a man who insanely thought his actions morally right should benefit from the defence; but since Windle's case in 1952[14] English courts have had to accept the doctrine that the Rules mean legal rightness. Windle's mentally ill wife talked persistently of suicide, and he became obsessed with this, bothering his workmates continually with the problem. One of them eventually said 'give her a dozen aspirins'. In the event he gave her a much larger dose than this, and killed her. His statement to the police made it clear that he knew he had committed a crime. (The nature of his mental illness – although this is hardly relevant – was described as *folie à deux*.) His defence failed to convince either the trial court or the Court of Criminal Appeal that his belief in the moral rightness of his action entitled him to an insanity verdict. Our doctrine is that only a belief that it was *legally* permissible to kill her would have excused him. In some jurisdictions belief that it was *morally* permissible would have succeeded, but that again is beside the point. The point is that the English courts were in effect preferring an interpretation which – though this was certainly not their reasoning – made mere possibility-explanations acceptable. A man who thinks it morally right to kill someone is under a stronger pressure to do so than a man who merely thinks it legally permissible. That sort of mistake about the law merely removes one good reason for *not* killing: it does not provide a good reason *for* killing. Windle's case neatly illustrates our courts' acceptance of mere possibility-explanations. Nor do I suggest that it did so *per incuriam*, for I am arguing that most of the excuses which courts accept from psychiatrists *do not assert that the defendant could not help it.*

Irresistible impulse

Automatism apart, it is only explanations of the 'irresistible impulse' sort which attempt to convince us that the defendant could not help it. Paradoxically, irresistible impulse is acceptable in Britain not as part of an insanity defence which excuses completely, but only as a basis for a defence of diminished responsibility.[15] The reason is the impossibility of knowing whether an impulse or desire was irresistible or just very hard or unpleasant to resist. Diminished responsibility allows us to settle for 'very hard to resist' without conceding that any impulse could be impossible to resist.

'Inexplicable' actions

Now and again one comes across cases of yet another sort, in which the psychiatrist frankly says that he cannot understand the subject's behaviour. This category is both the most controversial and the most interesting of all. It is controversial because some psychiatrists believe, while others refuse to believe, that unless behaviour is of the kind called automatism it is at least in theory intelligible. A psychiatrist who uses the notion of inexplicable actions says, in effect

(i) that the defendant was disordered when his action took place;
(ii) that the defendant has been able to talk to him about his state of mind at the time, but
(iii) that the action is nevertheless inexplicable; more precisely that even what he knows about the kind of disorder, plus what the accused has told him, does not enable him to make sense of the action.

No doubt some psychiatrists would dismiss such cases by saying that the psychiatrist in question has merely failed to communicate sufficiently with the accused, perhaps because the accused has too little insight, or too limited a vocabulary, perhaps because the psychiatrist lacks the special skill needed to talk to this sort of patient, perhaps because there is not time for a protracted series of interviews. Certainly we are very reluctant to entertain the notion of an intentional action that makes no sense at all, even in the distorted world of the mentally ill.

With the help of several psychiatrists I once tried to collect examples of criminal behaviour by disordered people which they found very hard to explain. One example was that of a young man who suddenly in a pub stabbed a girl whom he hardly knew, and who had not in any way provoked or sexually attracted him. He came from a stable harmonious family, had shown no behaviour problems, did not have a drinking problem, and had drunk only 'a pint or two'. But over the previous year he had been having a feeling of being possessed by an external force which ordered him to do evil things, although this seems to have been the first occasion on which he did anything serious.

Another case was that of a man in his sixties who was an inpatient in an ordinary National Health Service hospital, diagnosed as a paranoid schizophrenic. He walked down to a shop in the town one day, bought a knife and with it stabbed another patient, whom he knew by sight but with whom he had no quarrel and of whom he had no fear. When interviewed by a consultant psychiatrist about his offence he said that he felt he was a rather special person, but not understood at the hospital, and wanted to be sent to Broadmoor or Rampton: so he decided to kill someone.

In the first of these cases, the consultant who described it to me was clearly unable to regard the man's behaviour as intelligible. He could not, that is, tell the story in a way that would enable him to say 'Now I see why he did it, even if I wouldn't have myself.' In the other case the consultant did get a reason of sorts out of the patient: that he felt he was someone so special that he ought to be in Broadmoor or Rampton, and that killing another patient would achieve this. Interestingly, however, one very eminent psychiatrist with whom I discussed this case said that he could not regard this as reasoning which had really caused the patient to kill: it was probably a rationalisation of something that the patient himself could not understand. This psychiatrist was in effect saying that even if the patient succeeds in offering a reason, his action is not necessarily explicable in terms of reasons.

On the other hand there are psychiatrists who do not accept that a purposeful action cannot be rendered intelligible, at least in theory. Their position seems to be that if the psychiatrist has the time and the skill to establish rapport with the patient, is able to 'talk his language' both literally and metaphorically, and so long as the patient is not too inarticulate, the psychiatrist should be able to arrive at an account of the patient's behaviour which would lead him to say 'I see why he did it', without necessarily implying that he would have done it himself for the same reason.[16] In the case of the man who said that he wanted to get to Broadmoor, killing another patient was not an entirely senseless way of going about it. It was selfish and callous. One wonders whether he had tried asking for a transfer before killing. One says that one could never resort to this method of arranging a transfer oneself. But it is intelligible in its way.

I am not so sure about the patient who says that he sometimes feels he is being told to do evil things. To liken him to the soldier who acts under superior orders is probably misleading. It seems more likely that he is trying to describe, in the best way he can, some sort of compulsion. It may be that a psychoanalyst could tell us why he had the compulsion; but I would still want to ask the psychoanalyst whether his explanation if true would make the behaviour inevitable, highly probable or merely not impossible.

Mechanistic explanations of purposeful actions

Suppose, however, that we are faced with psychiatrists whose conclusion is that the defendant's action is inexplicable: that is, that they either cannot guess at his reasons or that they do not accept the reasons he gives. Are they implying that the subject was, during the crucial period, merely a machine? This implication could take one of two forms. They may be regarding him as a machine which was more or less bound to operate as he did. That would not be inconsistent with behaviour which seemed purposeful, like going to a shop for a knife before stabbing someone: machines can behave with apparent purpose.

Or they might mean that his movements were random, like those of machines such as Ernie,[17] or, at a simpler level, a roulette wheel. This would not merely mean that the 'choice' of victim was random: for that could happen in a crime by a non-disordered person, for example when hostages are taken on the spur of the moment. What is conceivably meant is that the defendant's behaviour was not even that of a 'purposeful' machine, but more like that of a machine which breaks down, or functions as it was not intended to, as a chess-playing computer does when it makes an illegal move.

It is for psychiatrists or neurologists, rather than me, to say what they think about my category of 'inexplicable' acts: whether it should be dismissed as a pseudo-category, created only by shortage of time, lack of expertise or the inarticulacy of the defendant, or whether, if it is a genuine category, it is made up of machine-like behaviour of a purposeful or random kind. There may even be some other analogy which is closer to what they mean, and which has not occurred to me.

Failing any agreement about, or further illumination of, this category, what view can courts take of it? Should it be accepted as automatism, insanity or diminished responsibility? It certainly ought not to qualify for a M'Naghten-type defence. An academic lawyer would probably be prepared to consider seriously whether it belongs to 'automatism'. A court would be unlikely to consider any defence other than diminished responsibility.

The infrequency of probability-explanations

Let me recapitulate the points made so far. The explanations which the law accepts from psychiatrists are, on the whole, merely possibility-explanations, and not usually probability-explanations, still less explanations in terms of inevitability. This shows why the text with which this paper began is nonsense. The questions which the M'Naghten Rules pose for psychiatrists have nothing to do with the presence or absence of free will. They are designed to discover whether, given the disordered person's strange view of reality, his actions were understandable, not inevitable.

What the authors of that text may have been expressing in a very loose way is the popular belief that the 'insane' criminal could not help what he did. In most cases, however, it seems closer to the facts to say that what he could not help was being disordered;[18] and that his disorder merely made his actions psychologically possible, not inevitable.

Paradoxically, it is diminished responsibility rather than M'Naghten-madness which allows courts to accept explanations of the kind that say, in effect, 'he was practically bound to do what he did in the circumstances'. At the other extreme of course, diminished responsibility admits explanations which merely say 'he was rather more likely than a person in an ordinary state of mind to do what he did'. In other words it is from the logical point of view a 'catch-all'.

It is only the defence of automatism which denies free will completely, by asserting that the defendant was moving like a machine. And even automatism does not necessarily imply the inevitability of the *actus reus*: often it is sheer bad luck that someone happened to be in the way of his movements. If, however, you believe in the category of inexplicable offences which I have been discussing, whether in the 'random behaviour' version of the 'purposeful machine' version, it really ought to be treated as automatism and not (as it seems to be in practice) as diminished responsibility.

The Butler Committee's proposals

English readers may be interested enough in this paper to wonder whether the Butler Committee's proposals for overhauling the psychiatric defences would, if implemented, make much difference so far as my specific point is conerned. But since (i) these proposals now seem unlikely to be enacted and (ii) they are of less interest to non-English readers, I have relegated them to Appendix 2, and will proceed to consider a solution which the Committee did not discuss but which might be of more interest to psychiatrists and lawyers from other common-law countries.

A simpler solution?

Could the Butler Committee have proposed something simpler? We could, although it would certainly have been rejected. What we could have recommended would have been the scrapping of everything but automatism and diminished responsibility, and the extension of diminished responsibility to any sort of offence, with one innovation. It has often been said that a conclusive objection to applying diminished responsibility to offences other than murder is that in most other cases there is no lesser legal category of offence to which the charge could be reduced. My suggestion – not the Butler Committee's, for we did not discuss this idea – is that the effect of diminished responsibility need not be a conviction of a less serious offence, but simply the mitigation, or better still the exclusion, of punitive measures. It could be enacted either that imprisonment, financial penalties and community service would be ruled out as a sentence, leaving commitment to hospital, psychiatric probation orders or discharges, absolute and conditional; or, less drastically, that a very restrictive limit should be set on the length of permissible prison sentence. Either of these versions would give the courts considerable discretion to choose a suitable disposal.

The exclusion of imprisonment would of course increase the pressure on hospitals to accept offenders whom they do not want; but that is a problem which exists already, and will have to be solved somehow. It may be asked whether the defendant would be convicted, and if not what the verdict should be. A possible answer is that it should be a 'finding of guilt' but not a conviction, as it is in juvenile courts. If it is objected that this is a distinction without much difference, I would have to concede this, but with the rider that the motto of the juvenile courts seems to be *vive la différence*.

Summary

If asked what I think I have been discussing here, I would have to reply that I have been covering some familiar ground in an unfamiliar way; trying to show that the usual defences based on mental disorder do not usually insist on deterministic explanations but merely on possibility-explanations of the kind we accept every day for the unexpected behaviour of ordinary people, the only important difference being the assumption that the defendant cannot help being disordered. I have suggested in Appendix 2 that the Butler proposals will avoid some problems, create some others, and probably deal in a rough but reasonable way with the problem of 'inexplicable' crimes by allowing them to qualify for the insanity defence. I have raised an old hare, the extension of diminished responsibility to offences other than homicide; but this time in a new form, which would remove the need for an insanity defence.

APPENDIX 1

A. The M'Naghten Rules (English version)

(i) The general test

'It must be clearly proved that, at the time of committing the act, the accused was labouring under such a defect of reason, from disease of the mind, as not to know the nature and quality of the act he was doing, or, if he did know it, that he did not know he was doing what was wrong.'

(ii) The relevance of delusions

'If a person under an insane delusion as to existing facts commits an offence in consequence thereof, is he thereby excused?'

'The answer must, of course, depend on the nature of the delusion; but making the same assumption as we did before, namely, that he labours under such partial delusion only, and is not in other respects insane, we think he must be considered in the same situation as to responsibility as if the facts with respect to which the delusion exists were real. For example, if under the influence of his delusion he supposes another man to be in the act of attempting to take away his life, and he kills that man, as he supposes, in self-defence, he would be exempt from punishment. If his delusion was that the deceased had inflicted a serious injury to his character and fortune, and he killed him in revenge for such supposed injury, he would be liable to punishment.'

Interpretation: 'wrong' means 'contrary to law'
In the Court of Criminal Appeal, in the case of Windle,[19] Lord Chief Justice Goddard said:

'Courts of law can only distinguish between that which is in accordance with the law and that which is contrary to law . . . The law cannot embark on the question and it would be an unfortunate thing if it were left to juries to consider whether some particular act was morally right or wrong. The test must be whether it is contrary to law'.

'In the opinion of the court there is no doubt that in the M'Naghten Rules "wrong" means contrary to law and not "wrong" according to the opinion of one man or of a number of people on the question whether a particular act might or might not be justified'.

B. Some American variants of the insanity defence

(i)   The 'Durham' Rule (propounded in Durham *v.* United States *(1954))*

'An accused is not criminally responsible if his unlawful act was the product of mental disease or mental defect.'[20]

(ii)   The American Law Institute's Model Clause of 1955

'(1) A person is not responsible for criminal conduct if at the time of such conduct as a result of mental disease or defect he lacks substantial capacity either to appreciate the criminality of his conduct or to conform his conduct to the requirements of law.

(2) As used in this Article, the terms 'mental disease or defect' do not include an abnormality manifested only by repeated criminal or otherwise antisocial conduct.'

(iii)   The 'Currens' Rule (propounded in United States *v.* Currens *(1961))*

'The jury must be satisfied that at the time of committing the prohibited act the defendant, as a result of mental disease or defect, lacked substantial capacity to conform his conduct to the requirements of the law which he is alleged to have violated.'

C. Diminished responsibility (Homicide Act 1957, s. 2(1))

'Where a person kills or is a party to the killing of another, he shall not be convicted of murder if he was suffering from such abnormality of mind (whether arising from a condition of arrested or retarded development of mind or any inherent causes or induced by disease or injury) as substantially impaired his mental responsibility for his acts and omissions in doing or being a party to the killing.'

Note the definition of 'abnormality of mind' given by the Lord Chief Justice (Lord Parker) in the Court of Criminal Appeal in the case of Byrne (1960):

'a state of mind so different from that of ordinary human beings that the reasonable man would term it abnormal. It appears to us to be wide enough to cover the mind's activities in all its aspects, not only the perception of physical acts and matters, and the ability to form a rational judgement as to whether the act was right or wrong, but also the ability to exercise will-power to control physical acts in accordance with that rational judgement.'

D. Infanticide (Infanticide Act 1938, s. 1)

'Where a woman by any wilful act or omission causes the death of her child under the age of twelve months, but at the time of the act or omission the balance of her mind was disturbed by reason of her not having fully recovered from the effect of giving birth to the child or by reason of the effect of lactation consequent upon the birth of the child, then, notwithstanding that the circumstances were such that but for this Act the offence would have amounted to murder, she shall be guilty of infanticide, and may for such offences be dealt with and punished as if she had been guilty of the offence of manslaughter of the child.'

E. Automatism

There is no statutory definition of this common-law defence. So far as case-law is concerned, it has been described as 'a modern catchphrase which the courts have not accepted as connoting any wider or looser concept than involuntary movement of the body or limbs or a person' (*Watmore* v. *Jenkins* [1962] 2 All ER at 874). It has succeeded in cases of somnambulism, hypoglycaemia, cerebral tumour, epilepsy and cerebral arteriosclerosis.

APPENDIX 2. The Butler Committee proposals

The relevant proposals of the Butler Committee[21] were:
1. that the defence of diminished responsibility should be abolished, but only if judges were given more freedom when sentencing persons convicted of murder;
2. that there should be two kinds of insanity defence:
   (i) based on the ground that the defendant's mental disorder resulted in his not having the 'state of mind required for the offence' (for example the specific intent which the definition of some crimes requires);
   (ii) based simply on the ground that at the time of his act or omission the defendant was suffering from severe mental illness or severe subnormality;
   and that after a successful insanity defence the court should be free to dispose of the defendant in non-custodial ways as well as by hospital orders;
3. that the defence of infanticide should be abolished and the prosecution allowed to charge manslaughter by reason of mental disorder;
4. that the defence of non-insane automatism, leading to an unqualified acquittal, should be retained, to cover transient states such as somnambulism.

The second version of the insanity defence – which is much wider in scope than the first, and much more likely to be used – would certainly make it unnecessary to ask psychiatrists awkward questions about the defendant's precise state of mind at the time of his *actus reus*. The only difficulty likely to arise is over the borderline between severe and non-severe disorder: but the Butler Committee provided guide-lines to reduce the difficulty.

In this form the insanity defence would accommodate the psychiatrist who finds the defendant's behaviour inexplicable, or who wants to say simply that a severely paranoid schizophrenic is very likely to do what the defendant did.

On the other hand, it must be realised that if diminished responsibility is abolished, there will be no place for the non-severe mental disorder which did not deprive the offender of the state of mind essential for a conviction of murder. Most psychopathic killers will just have to be convicted of murder. Some might welcome that; others may be relieved to know that diminished responsibility will almost certainly not be abolished, since the penalty for murder is now most unlikely to be made discretionary.

(By contrast, the first version of the Butler insanity defence *would* make it necessary to put very precise questions to psychiatrists, of a kind which – in my own personal view – they could answer only with spurious precision.)

The retention of non-insane automatism, in the form recommended by the Butler Committee, would not allow acquittals in 'inexplicable' cases in which the inexplicable behaviour was apparently associated with persistent or recurrent mental disorder. These would come under the second version of the new insanity defence, and not, as at present, under diminished responsibility. From the point of view of the protection of others it is clearly undesirable that they should lead to unqualified acquittals with no possibility of precautionary measures under a court order; and from the point of view of justice it seems preferable that they should qualify for a special verdict rather than be stigmatised as manslaughter.

NOTES

1. For the legal wording used to define the various 'psychiatric defences', see Appendix 1.
2. See note 4.
3. W.H. Dray *Laws and Explanations in History* (1957, Oxford University Press).
4. *Behaviour and Misbehaviour: explanations and non-explanations* (1977, Blackwell, Oxford).
5. M. Scriven, 'Explanations, prediction and laws', *Minnesota Studies in the Philosophy of Science*, ed. R. Feigl, 3 (1962), 190ff.
6. E.g. Sir Alfred Ayer, 'Man as a subject of science', in *Philosophy, Politics and Society*, ed. P. Laslett and W. Runciman (1967, Blackwell, Oxford).
7. Or indeed any other conduct, so long as it is *unexpected*. We don't ask psychiatrists to explain everyday behaviour.
8. The distinction between sane and non-insane automatism seems irrelevant in this context.
9. W. Böker and H. Häfner, *Gewalttäten Geistesgestorter* (1973, Springer-Verlag,

Berlin). I have relied on the English summary by the authors in *Social Psychiatry*, 8 (1973), 220ff.

10. I know that for many psychiatrists such addictions are not 'mental disorders', but in the present context this is not relevant: we expect psychiatrists to help in explaining the behaviour associated with them.

11. B. Wootton *Social Science and Social Pathology* (1959, Allen & Unwin, London). I have argued in *Crime and Insanity in England*, vol. II, ed. N. Walker and S. McCabe (1973, Edinburgh University Press) that although 'psychopathy' has hardly enough descriptive, prognostic or other utility to entitle it to the status of a diagnosis, it is not quite as 'circular' an explanation as Lady Wootton suggests.

12. In fact, this may be an advantage. An imaginary case is likely to be a purer illustration of what the imaginer is getting at than a case which is complicated by reality.

13. *R. v. Male* (1964) unreported: but see the account in my *Crime and Insanity in England*, vol. I (1968, Edinburgh University Press), p. 118. It would be plausible to say that a lasting delusion of this sort would make him likely to steal food. This chronic sort of mistake is a better basis for a probability-explanation than a mistake as to the nature and quality of one's act. But even if it had been a transient delusion it would still have been a sound basis for an insanity defence. Again, it does not seem that the defence demands that the disease of the mind make the action probable. If the *soi-disant* prophet had had money in his pocket he might well have paid for the food.

14. [1952] 2 QB 826 CCA.

15. Nor are there many common-law jurisdictions where it does figure in the insanity defence. The usual North American addition to M'Naghten type rules is not irresistible impulse but lack of the capacity to conform to the requirements of the law: i.e. not a compelling reason *for* doing something but an inability to restrain oneself if one wants to but knows it to be criminal: another example of a possibility-explanation.

16. This seems also to be the position of Professor D. Cressey, *Delinquency, Crime and Differential Association* (1964, Nijhoff, The Hague), chapter VI. This chapter, however, does little more than assert this view, without adducing evidence.

17. The British computer which chooses winning numbers of Premium Bonds.

18. Except in the rare case in which he contributed to his disorder by voluntarily taking alcohol or drugs.

19. [1952] 2 QB 826; 2 All ER 1.

20. Note the resemblance to the New Hampshire direction to the jury (in 1869) in which the term 'product' was used:
    'Neither delusion nor knowledge of right and wrong, nor design or cunning in planning and executing the killing and escaping or avoiding detection, nor ability to recognise acquaintances, or to labour or transact business or manage affairs, is, as a matter of law, a test of mental disease; but . . . all symptoms and all tests of mental disease are purely matters of fact, to be determined by the jury . . . Whether the defendant had a mental disease, and whether the killing of his wife was the product of such disease, are questions of fact for the jury.'

21. *Report of the Committee on Mentally Abnormal Offenders* (Chairman: Lord Butler) 1975: Cmnd 6244. London, HMSO.

Detention of patients: administrative problems facing Mental Health Review Tribunals

SIR JOHN WOOD

Introduction

The recent reforms now embodied in the Mental Health Act 1983 are the culmination of pressure to improve the legal rights of patients and to protect and enforce those rights effectively. The emphasis upon the part to be played by the law is clear from the publications of MIND (see Gostin 1975, 1977).[1] The very process of securing the reforms has swung attention to the process of legislation and its detailed form. Doctors discussing the changes come to sound like lawyers. American experience, with its much greater emphasis on legal control, is greatly relied upon. The traditional English dependence upon professional standards and sound but humane administration is seriously questioned. The occasional 'error' or 'scandal' is used to justify the need for greater legal control.

Of course this is not true for all of the reforms. One of the most important, the Mental Health Act Commission, builds firmly on regulation by fellow professionals.[2] This should be, in the long run, the most important of the many reforms because it has a role much wider than the misfortunes or dissatisfaction of an individual patient. On the other hand there has also been a considerable strengthening of the Mental Health Review Tribunals, the subject of this paper. They have represented, since the Mental Health Act 1959, the impact of legal challenge upon one aspect of medical discretion, the right to detain. It was inevitable that they would be used to improve the legal protection of the detained patient.

It is not necessary to set out the legal changes in detail. Attention has to be paid both to the 1983 Act and to the revised rules of procedure,[3] both of which came into force at the beginning of October 1983. The most obvious change is the doubling of the opportunity to apply to a tribunal which in general terms will be annual. Equally important is the duty of the detaining authority itself to refer a patient to a tribunal after 3 years if there has been no application. The rules seek to make the act of application easier and less formal, to improve the flow of information to the tribunal, the patient and his representative and to give a more standardised form to the actual proceedings.

The need for standardisation is itself significant since it springs from a dual perception of the role of the tribunal. To many the tribunal is precisely what its name suggests, a review of the need for detention made by an independent group of mixed disciplines (lawyers, psychiatrists, laymen). The form of the proceedings has many of the characteristics of a court of law, but the function differs. It is not, in this view, adversarial but investigatory. Others stress the adversarial aspect. They cast the patient in the role of complainant–plaintiff and the detaining authority as the defendant. This approach emphasises the role of the responsible medical officer (invariably referred to as RMO). He becomes in effect not merely chief source of evidence; his role tends to resemble that of a party to the proceedings. It would appear that the first of these views still predominates. If it failed to do so the legalisation of the process would need special attention, for unless it was carefully controlled it would be destructive of the RMO–patient relationship and even perhaps of the overall relationship of hospital to patients in general.

It is the thesis of this paper that the strengthening of the legal framework protecting the patient will be relatively ineffective unless it is matched by parallel administrative changes. Most reformers feel, erroneously, that once they have secured 'their' legislation the battle has been won. But it is rarely so. Not only is there often a reactionary response which, by counter-moves, subverts at least in part the aims of the legislation, but also prevailing attitudes and administrative procedures (which cannot be changed by mere legislation) seem obstinately unable to accommodate the changes. There is real evidence that in the case of detained patients the obstacles will prove to be very weighty indeed. It is a fear that needs urgent discussion. First it is necessary to look at the powers of detention and release.

Detention and release

Two types of detention must be distinguished: civil and criminal. In general terms the former arises where patients are detained on medical advice, the latter where the courts, having found a person guilty of crime, commit them to hospital, again after taking medical advice. The system is not of course as tidy as that. Some criminals are transferred to hospital from prison. Some charged with crime and found unfit to stand trial are detained in hospital. For the purpose of this discussion the important distinction lies within criminal detention.

This is because in all cases but one (ignoring the special 'hold until fit to stand trial') the RMO can discharge the order allowing detention. That important distinction is where the court has added to the order a restriction. This may be for a stated period or specified 'without limit in time'. In respect of those patients the detention has been controlled by the Home Office.

That has meant that Mental Health Review Tribunals have dealt with two distinct types of case. Applications have been made by those under civil (usually s.26 of the 1959 Act) or criminal detention (s.60 of the 1959 Act) and references from the Home Office regarding those in criminal detention and covered by a restriction (s.65 of the 1959 Act provided for the restriction). The cases were significantly different in that in respect of the former group the tribunal had power to discharge, while in respect of the latter it had to recommend, to the Home Office, the appropriate course of action.

It was a system with a central paradox. Where it had power the tribunal had only one choice – to release or not. Where its function was restricted to advice it could recommend a variety of actions – conditional discharge, home leave, transfer from secure to open hospital – with no certainty that its advice would be heeded. The obvious reform, from the standpoint of the tribunal, was at least the granting of wider powers in those cases where it could make an enforceable order. It is ironic that the real reform has come in the other group.

The reason lies outside the basic reforms. The failure of the existing law to give the restricted patient the right to an independent judicial review was challenged in the European Court at Strasbourg.[4] The point was upheld by the court so changes were made in the legislation to meet this objection.

The new powers of tribunals can be briefly summarised. They are all based upon a revised set of criteria (previously s.123, 1959 Act: now s.72, 1983 Act). The tribunal *must* discharge a patient who does not fall within the four categories justifying detention[5] or who need not be detained to secure his own health or safety or the protection of others. In making that decision the tribunal must look at the likelihood of treatment alleviating or preventing a deterioration of the patient's condition and must also assess how far a mentally ill or severely mentally impaired patient could care for himself or obtain the necessary help. In addition to these powers the tribunal may direct discharge at a future date. It can also recommend to the authorities leave of absence, or transfer to another hospital or into guardianship, and can reconvene at a later date if such action is not taken.

It will be seen that apart from the deferred discharge, the powers of the tribunal have been extended only in the form of recommendations. This is perhaps the central reason why administrative action remains of crucial importance.

In respect of restricted patients the powers are clearer: to discharge absolutely or conditionally in appropriate cases (s.73, 1983 Act). This power, which will apply to many very serious criminals, has led to a restructuring of tribunals for such cases. The legal president in restricted cases must be either a circuit judge or a silk recorder, that is to say a person who has had experience in sentencing criminals. This is a nice example of an administrative change – it is not difficult to see its purposes. There are, however, very many obstacles to thwart the liberal intentions of those who have pressed for legislative change.

Obstacles to change

The reforms have reached the statute book at precisely the time when the Government is faced with economic difficulties. Even leaving aside the increasingly strident arguments about cutting services, it is obvious that in most developed countries some restraint upon the growth of public expenditure on the social services is likely to be imposed. Ironically the implementation of a liberal attitude to detention of mental patients should be a saving. It will not be so, however, at the outset when capital spending is needed on new institutions such as intermediate secure hospitals, hostels and day care centres. Above all the perceived shortage of resources allows those in charge of the movement of patients to discriminate against the marginal case. Thus the patient in a Special Hospital (that is one with strict security) can be turned down by an open hospital 'for lack of resources', a reason that may conceal an underlying unwillingness to shoulder yet another difficult newcomer.

It is also important to note that the public attitude to the movement of patients is a powerful factor. As far as the press is concerned, a tribunal decision can be open to criticism without difficulty. A patient who continues to be detained may be able to win sympathy, especially if the ostensible cause of detention can be made to appear to be a youthful indiscretion. The authorities, who no doubt have argued over the decision to continue detention, except in rare cases, can be made to look heartless. A discharge, on the other hand, must involve the tribunal 'overruling the RMO', this showing, it is suggested, its careless and cavalier approach to danger to the public. Such treatment can be applied to decisions at every level. The result is to encourage a safety-first approach.

The underlying aim of the legislation and its implementation needs to be made clearer. It is a defect of the legislative process that it uses technical legal language and fails to record the aims. Even the Victorian long title to a statute has been dropped. So it is necessary to search through the speeches in Parliament, which are soon forgotten, to give the real context of legislation. That of the aspects of the mental health legislation being discussed is clear. It is to ensure as far as is possible that a patient enjoys the maximum amount of freedom consistent with his own health and safety and the protection of others. All the institutions should have this as their fundamental aim. Often they do not appear to do so.

The Government

Two departments of state, the Home Office and the Department of Health and Social Security (DHSS), have responsibility for detained patients. The former has responsibility for restricted patients, the latter for all patients. The discharge of those responsibilities is best exercised in respect of the transfer of patients from Special Hospitals to open hospitals. It is a topic which has been aired in part in 1980 by a Special Hospitals Research Report.[6] It is only necessary to point to two aspects of practice to indicate the difficulties.

Where a tribunal made a recommendation to the Home Office under the system just superseded, the first step was to ask the RMO his views. It became obvious from the length of time taken before a decision on the recommendation was made in many cases – it could be as long as two years – that the work of the tribunal was regarded as an indicator that investigations should begin rather than that transfer should be seriously considered. The reason for the caution is clear. The Home Office is concerned primarily with public safety. Its concept of failure must be the transfer that goes wrong: at its most grim the released murderer who murders again. That is understandable, but unless the impossibility of a risk-free transfer is accepted it leads to a restrictive and conservative policy. Certainly that appears to have been the pattern in the period 1959– 1983.

It is only necessary to look at the Report mentioned above[6] and to recall that restricted patients accepted as suitable for transfer by the Home Office may remain for several years longer in the Special Hospitals – two to six years is not uncommon – to realise that the DHSS cannot be said to have pursued an actively liberal policy. Indeed the final sentences of the Report can be used as evidence of this:

> A worrying feature of the present position is that although the Department [DHSS] is responsible for both the National Health Service and the Special Hospitals, it behaves as though it were unaware of this. When questions are asked in Parliament about

the long delays in transfer, Ministers have simply regretted and deplored them (e.g. Hansard, 1977).[7] Consequently national policy is made by default, and transfers in some cases have become unobtainable – a wait of eight years means nothing else. The time has come for the responsible Department to accept responsibility.

If policy goes by default, practice arises from a number of ingrained attitudes. It is to these we must now give attention.

Medical and nursing professions

It is ironic, but alas true, that the caring professions themselves can pose obstacles to a patient. At its best this springs from the difficulty of balancing the need for care and control with as much freedom as is possible. The special features of psychiatry have led to the acceptance that no psychiatrist should have a patient assigned to his care without the patient's consent.

Where transfer between hospitals is in question the tensions and problems become clear. A Special Hospital, satisfied that a patient is ready for more freedom, has the task of getting the patient 'accepted'. A Mental Health Review Tribunal, exercising its judgment, finds this task very hard indeed. The new provisions, which envisage its making a recommendation, are likely, unless things change remarkably, merely to underline where power really lies.

Indeed several factors appear to be adding to the difficulties. Shortage of resources must be mentioned again. It is also important to note that the practice of zoning means that a patient's consultant-to-be may be precisely determined by his place of residence. This tends to give the individual consultant a powerful right of veto.

This right appears also to be vested in the consultant's nursing staff. Obviously it is right that the views of nurses who will have the patient in their care should be taken into account. That this should be taken as the right to a permanent veto on transfer is less defensible. Yet it is an important feature of the current scene. In a slightly different context, the admission of patients from court under s.60 (now s.3) has been also subject to veto by nurses and has led to a sharply worded judgment from Lord Justice Lawton.[8] If the patient in a Special Hospital was transferred there some years previously because of behaviour that could not be contained it is difficult to expect a welcome return.

The difficulty, however, is made worse because of administrative problems, common to so many areas. For example acceptance would be easier if it were on a probationary basis. Such flexibility is hard to arrange.

Indeed difficulties increase. The shortage of resources has led certain consultants to accept patients only if the next stage, e.g. a hostel, is arranged at the outset. This has been the policy at Eastdale[9] for the simple reason that a short-stay hospital/hostel could not cope with a 'bow wave' of patients. But the difficulty of securing a future placement, at best difficult, becomes increasingly so. It is the patient who suffers. Care, whether under order or voluntary, can only be regarded as a contract. If the patient does what is asked of him he is surely entitled to the level of care and freedom earned, and a system which administratively denies him this is grossly unfair.

Local authorities and community care

The pressure on resources is perhaps even more keenly felt at the level of community care, so again must be mentioned first. An excerpt from a Home Circumstances Report recently received by the Trent Mental Health Review Tribunal fully makes the point:

> [The County] accepts that it has some financial and moral obligation to help resettle [the patient] back into the community. However, we have few suitable resources. We do support clients in private or voluntary hostels, but we have a waiting list of over 100 mental health clients – as you are aware our money is allocated on a 'head count' basis. This means, realistically, that [the patient] will be waiting indefinitely for financial help.

That such a passage has to occur in a report otherwise showing exemplary concern and willingness to help could not be a clearer indication of malaise.

But again there are other difficulties. There appears to be little co-ordination between the hospitals in general and local authority social services. It is very rare to find the necessary preliminary co-ordination between community psychiatrist services and other services, a defect springing directly from the distinct administrative boxes of 'health' and 'social services'.

It is difficult to integrate these existing difficulties into the often-made assertion that the future pattern of care of the mentally disabled will be based on community care. This is likely to require a great deal of improvement in the present administrative arrangements. It is too often forgotten that one of the principal functions of hospital or sheltered hostel is well described by the now unfashionable word 'asylum'.

Administrative obstacles

It is sad that reformers tend to overlook the administrative aspects of change. Although a change in the law will inevitably ensure change it will not be very effective unless those responsible for the implementation of the new rules wish them to succeed. Even then success will be harmed if the necessary resources do not follow the change.

Restricted patients, following the European Court decision in 1981, should have greater chance of gaining their freedom when this is indicated. All the signs are that despite the changes in the 1983 Act they will not benefit and may well suffer. This arises from several factors:

1. Attitudes in society appear to be changing. The failure of the capital punishment lobby to secure its return has led to a tightening in the 'effectiveness' of long sentences. This will inevitably make harder the task of allowing a mental patient to gain greater freedom quicker. Yet the aim of the legislation was to tackle those remaining in custody when medical opinion held the risk of release or transfer acceptable.

2. Shortages of resources, of purpose-built secure hospitals, of staff, of community care, will add a further burden. It will inevitably enable those whose approach is one of extreme caution to justify very restrictive responses.

3. The restructuring of the Mental Health Review Tribunals to ensure that the president is a judge or recorder with current sentencing experience can only be regarded as an over-emphasis on the public safety aspect of the problem.

4. The failure to give those reconstructed tribunals a clear power to transfer (e.g. to local hospital or hostel) shows a reluctance to give the reform teeth.

Other patients will find too that the idealist aim of adequate community care is not readily available. This is not to blame those offering care. They find the pressures of a more liberal process of release from detention an added burden. Is it fair to give them a stable schizophrenic, for example, 'in the hope that this time stability can be found in the community'? There is so much else that is important and perhaps more rewarding.

In the ultimate much of what has been said here need not take place. But the demand for changes in attitude is a severe one and only a true optimist can feel confident that they will take place.

NOTES

1. *A Human Condition*, vols. 1 and 2. National Association for Mental Health, London.
2. See Mental Health Act 1983, s.121.
3. The Mental Health Review Tribunal Rules 1983 – SI 1983/942.
4. *X*. v. *United Kingdom*, 5 November 1981, European Court of Human Rights.
5. Mental Illness, psychopathic disorder, severe mental impairment, mental impairment.
6. No. 16. The Transfer of Special Hospital Patients to National Health Service Hospitals. Susanne Dell.
7. 16 June 77, vol. 933, col. 266.
8. *R*. v. *Harding* [1983], Law Report, *The Times* 15 June.
9. A hospital at Newark, specially designed as a step (six months) between special hospital and the community.

Developments in forensic psychiatry services in the National Health Service

JOHN R. HAMILTON*

This paper aims to describe the present state of forensic psychiatry services in the United Kingdom. These services can be divided into those provided by Special Hospitals for the whole country by the Department of Health and Social Security (DHSS), and secure units and community forensic psychiatry services provided by the National Health Service (NHS) regions. Only passing reference is made to the Prison Medical Service, as that is covered in the following chapter by Professor Gunn.

Special Hospitals

Many incorrectly believe forensic psychiatry to be a fairly new specialty within the profession, whereas it is of the same age as general psychiatry in terms of the provision of institutional facilities. The national system of mental hospitals originated in the County Asylums Act of 1808 and the provision of special facilities for mentally abnormal offenders can be dated from the year 1800 when a paranoid schizophrenic, James Hadfield, was found not guilty by reason of insanity of shooting at King George III. At his trial the judge commented: 'this unfortunate man should be cared for, all mercy and humanity being shown'. Hadfield was committed to the long-established Bethlem Hospital in London which had added to it a criminal wing, and to ensure his legal detention the first Criminal Lunatics Act was passed to cater for those acquitted on the grounds of insanity or found insane on arraignment and ordered to be detained in custody 'until His Majesty's Pleasure be known'.

Over the next 60 years many other criminal lunatics accumulated in the Bethlem and in other hospitals and prisons, causing penal reformists such as Shaftesbury to criticise the mixing together of criminals and lunatics. A

---

* The views expressed are the author's own and are not necessarily those of the Department of Health and Social Security.

Select Committee of the House of Commons reported in 1860 that such mixing was 'a serious evil' and in the same year the second Criminal Lunatics Act was passed with the purpose of making better provision for their custody and care, and authorising the building of a Criminal Lunatics Asylum for them. In 1863 Broadmoor opened, the oldest of the Special Hospitals, under the management of the Home Office. (For the history of Broadmoor see Partridge (1953) and Hamilton (1980).) Criminal lunatics were transferred to Broadmoor from the Bethlem and other establishments throughout the country, but by the turn of the century the hospital was badly overcrowded and a decision was taken to open a new criminal lunatic asylum, Rampton, to fulfil the same functions as Broadmoor. Rampton opened in 1910. In 1920 its management passed to the Board of Control under the Mental Deficiency Act 1913 to cater for mental defectives of dangerous and violent propensities. Until 1960 patients could only be admitted to Rampton under the Mental Deficiency Acts and most were transferred to Rampton from other hospitals whether or not they had previously faced criminal charges.

By 1933 it was necessary to open a further state institution for mental defectives, and Moss Side opened with 400 beds. By the late 1950s Broadmoor had again become seriously overcrowded and Park Lane, next to Moss Side, opened with an Advance Unit in 1974. Most of Park Lane's current patients have been transferred from Broadmoor.

In Scotland the State Hospital, Carstairs, was opened in 1948 for the admission of mental defectives and in 1957 for those suffering from mental illness, the patients being transferred from the criminal lunatic department of Perth Prison. In Scotland, then, the State Hospital takes patients with varied forms of mental disorder, but in England the situation has been different.

Broadmoor and Park Lane have virtually no patients with mental handicap: in both these hospitals the patient populations are roughly 75% mental illness and 25% psychopathic disorder. Although Rampton and Moss Side were intended to treat only mentally handicapped patients the situation has changed (without any particular policy intending this) over the years, so that at present only a minority of patients in each of these hospitals has a Mental Health Act 1983 classification of mental impairment or severe mental impairment; there are large numbers of patients with both mental illness and psychopathic disorder though the nursing staff are by and large still only trained in mental handicap nursing. There are differences too in the legal categories of detention in the different English Special Hospitals. Whilst in Broadmoor and Park Lane 80% of the patients are under restriction orders, in Rampton and Moss Side there are equal numbers of unrestricted and restricted patients.

Patients cannot be admitted to Special Hospitals from the courts or elsewhere unless a bed has been made available for them. Whereas in Scotland the decision whether or not to accept a patient is the responsibility of the Physician Superintendent of the State Hospital, in England at the present time such decisions are made by a team of civil servants in the mental health branch of the DHSS in London. The majority of patients, however, are also seen by a Special Hospital consultant who advises on the suitability of admission.

Overall in the Special Hospitals roughly 60% of the patients have been made subject to hospital orders following conviction for serious offences in the courts, 20% have been transferred from other psychiatric hospitals and are on civil commitment orders, and 10% are patients who have been transferred from prison while serving a sentence. Smaller groups are detained under other provisions of the Mental Health Act 1983 and the Criminal Procedure (Insanity) Act 1964.

There has been in recent years a fall in the number of patients transferred from prison to Special Hospitals. Whilst at the latest 'census' only 68 prisoners serving sentence were thought by prison medical officers to be suffering from mental illness which warranted admission to hospital, many psychiatrists believe that this is a gross under-estimate. It is believed there are many others who have not been recorded as suffering from mental illness because prison medical officers (on the basis of their past experiences) have thought they were unlikely to succeed in effecting transfer to hospitals. Of the total number, whatever it might be, there is no indication how many should be in the conditions of special security of a Special Hospital, in a regional or interim secure unit or simply in an ordinary NHS psychiatric hospital. The proportion of prisoners transferred to Special Hospitals rather than NHS hospitals has risen from 25% in 1966 to 42% in 1981, in that year there being a total of 86 prisoners transferred. On the other hand only a very small number of patients found under disability in relation to trial (unfit to plead) are admitted to Special Hospitals: in 1981 26 of the 33 such cases were admitted to local hospitals.

The number of admissions to Special Hospitals each year is roughly half the number of applications for admission. Two out of three applications for the mentally ill are successful, the mentally subnormal (under the 1959 Act) had a one in three chance of being accepted and those with psychopathic disorder and the very few severely subnormal patients had an even chance. The number of applications received since 1977 (about 350 each year) has dropped markedly from the level in the early 1970s when about 500 applications were made each year. The acceptance rate has remained steady over the last 5 years at about 300 per annum and there has consequently been a drop in the last 2 years in the number rejected. The probable explanation is that those likely to be rejected are not having applications made for them.

The total number of patients in the Special Hospitals has been falling steadily over the last 15 years. In 1968 there were 2500 patients in the three English Special Hospitals and the State Hospital. In mid-1984 patient distribution numbers between the Special Hospitals were: Broadmoor 550, Rampton 600, Moss Side 250 and Park Lane 250, and the population of the State Hospital Carstairs had decreased to about 280. The fall in the number of patients in Rampton from 900 a few years ago to the current 600 was helped largely by the transfer of a large number of patients who had been waiting for transfer until the implementation of the findings of Susanne Dell's (1980) report. In June 1983, however, the Special Hospitals still had 248 patients (1 in 7 of the resident population) awaiting transfer or conditional discharge.

Broadmoor Hospital is having its 120-year-old buildings gradually demolished and over the next 15 years a new purpose-built hospital will be completed (NHS funding permitting) with a total of about 500 beds. Park Lane is due for completion in 1985, at which time it will have about 400 beds. At this time the Special Hospitals will have a maximum of about 1700 to 1800 patients, which is a reduction of perhaps 25% on the figures two years ago.

It is interesting to note that Scotland has maintained a tradition of 'consuming its own smoke', with each psychiatric hospital maintaining a locked ward for disturbed patients. There are no plans for regional secure units in Scotland but the provision of beds in the State Hospital Carstairs is approximately 50% higher per capita than that for England and Wales.

In England there has been a change in attitude of psychiatric staff towards mentally abnormal offenders and disturbed patients since 1960. Before then there was a considerable degree of expertise among nursing and medical staff in handling dangerous and violent patients. The coming into force of the Mental Health Act 1959, however, led to the development of 'open door' philosophies which were taken literally, with doors being unlocked and the keys thrown away; with them went the ability and willingness to handle such patients. Matters were perhaps not helped either by the new Act allowing patients to be transferred to Special Hospitals on civil commitment orders without the necessity for conviction in the courts. Others, however, take the view that this has contributed towards more open regimes in psychiatric hospitals and a greater willingness on the part of the public to use the psychiatric services.

Special Hospitals have always been favourite targets for the media and civil rights bodies, being condemned either for keeping patients too long or for discharging them too soon. The small and perhaps inevitable recidivism rate has to be examined alongside the fact that Special Hospitals discharge each year as many patients as they admit and at any one time there are thousands of ex-Special Hospital patients successfully rehabilitated in the community.

Criticisms that have been levelled against the Special Hospitals in the past, such as an inadequate complaints procedure, the use of seclusion and treatment without consent, should be resolved by the new mental health legislation (see Bluglass, this volume). The Mental Health Act 1983 awards patients greater rights and makes their position on consent to treatment clear. Criteria for detention and renewal of detention have been tightened together with an essential 'treatability' criterion for psychopathic disorder (and mental impairment). Access to Mental Health Review Tribunals for appeal against detention has been increased, though as a result Special Hospital psychiatrists will have to spend an increasing amount of time justifying detention at the expense of time spent treating patients.

The provisions in the new Mental Health Act for the making of interim hospital orders and providing for remands for assessment and for treatment will also provide new exciting opportunities for staff as well as for research and teaching purposes. The Government announced the implementation of these proposals from October 1984. Finally the new Mental Health Act Commission proposes to visit Special Hospitals on a regular basis and will in time provide a necessary safety valve for patients as the Mental Welfare Commission does in Scotland.

Future of Special Hospitals

The reduction in the number of patients in Special Hospitals and the growth of NHS secure facilities have led some to question the need for Special Hospitals to continue, but the general view is that it is too early to forecast how forensic services will develop.

The Royal College of Psychiatrists (1980) in its report on secure facilities stated:

> The Special Hospitals are situated at one end of the range of secure treatment facilities and should be closely integrated operationally with them. They will continue to provide conditions of maximum security for those exhibiting dangerous, violent or criminal propensities and also requiring special security, as they do at the present time. The College envisages movement between the Special Hospitals and other types of Unit, facilitated by close working co-operation and dependent

upon the degree of security and intensive care made necessary by the patient's psychiatric disorder and behaviour.

In its policy statement *The Future of Special Hospitals* (and the State Hospital) the College (Royal College of Psychiatrists, 1983) declared itself still in favour of the retention of Special Hospitals, noting that neither the Butler Committee nor any authoritative report has advocated doing away with them:

> It is clear that Regional Secure Units will only be able to function effectively with patients who do not need treatment in conditions of maximum security. For other patients Special Hospitals will still be required and they have advantages of providing a range of facilities appropriate for patients requiring a prolonged stay in hospital.
>
> . . .
>
> The national provision of secure facilities for psychiatric patients requires the continuation of maximum security Special Hospitals. They are necessary for patients whose dangerousness and length of treatment required are such as to make them unsuitable for smaller regional and local secure facilities, but there should be a close integration and flexible operational arrangements between all types of facilities.

The College's report examined many aspects of the work of Special Hospitals and the State Hospital. On management the College recommended the establishment of a local management committee where that was wanted or necessary, though it recognised there would be disadvantages were such a structure to be imposed on a well-functioning hospital. Security was thought to be satisfactory though a balance had to be struck between the degree of security necessary for the protection of the public and the amount necessary to enable treatment to be effective.

The College deplored the continued existence in Special Hospitals of patients who no longer required maximum security: 'the development of local secure facilities is essential to cut this to a minimum'.

Secure units

With the coming into force of the 1959 Act the Ministry of Health set up a working party to consider the role of the Special Hospitals; their report (Ministry of Health, 1961) said that security arrangements should continue to be provided in some regional NHS hospitals as well as in 'special diagnostic centres' for patients who presented difficult assessment and treatment problems. These centres would be important in research, provide an intermediate function between the NHS and Special

Hospitals and be financed directly by the Ministry though under local health service management. Only one such clinic in fact opened, the Northgate Clinic in London, which soon afterwards became a specialised adolescent unit.

In 1972 the Butler Committee on mentally abnormal offenders was established and in 1974 was so concerned (Home Office and Department of Health and Social Security, 1974) at overcrowding in Special Hospitals that it issued an interim report recommending the setting up of regional secure units to fill what it called the 'yawning gap' between Special Hospitals and NHS hospitals; the initial target was 2000 secure places. At about the same time the DHSS set up a working party on security in NHS psychiatric hospitals chaired by Dr J. Glancy (Department of Health and Social Security, 1974) which recommended that 1000 secure beds should be provided in secure accommodation in NHS hospitals. The Government accepted the recommendations of both Committees and made available direct financial assistance to set up interim security arrangements, the 'interim' meaning temporary (although others have interpreted this as meaning a degree of security mid-way between that provided in Special Hospitals and that of a locked ward).

In 1975 the Butler Committee (Home Office and Department of Health and Social Security, 1975) expressed their concern that so little progress had been made in establishing the units, but in the subsequent 5 years little more was achieved. Parliamentary questions were frequently tabled and the Royal College of Psychiatrists set up a special committee under the chairmanship of Professor R. Bluglass which made detailed recommendations on the establishment of regional and sub-regional units as well as secure units in psychiatric hospitals. The report (Royal College of Psychiatrists, 1980), as mentioned above, emphasised the need for flexibility, with facilities appropriate to local needs and integration of the forensic psychiatry services in each region. The level of secure provision would range from that in the open-door hospital at the one end, to the Special Hospitals at the other, with free movement of patients between the facilities according to their need.

Future of secure units

The current position of regional secure unit development has recently been comprehensively reviewed by Snowden (1985). At the end of 1984 there were seven permanent regional secure units admitting patients in Middlesborough, Dawlish, Leicester, Liverpool, Norwich, Wakefield and Southend. Units in other regions, including a multi-site scheme in South-East Thames, were nearing completion. Four further regional units were at various planning stages. In the meantime the prestigious pioneering work in the interim units particularly in Knowle, Rainhill and Prestwich has provided valuable information on the types of patients who can and cannot be managed in these units. Currently there are about 260 places available in 15 interim secure units, and discussions continue as to whether or how these units will be used when the regional units are completed. More information should be available soon from a research study on the operation of secure units being conducted by Professor Gwynne Jones at the Forensic Psychiatry Department in Birmingham.

Staff in Special Hospitals, however, remain sceptical as to how the new units will assist them in either taking patients on transfer or preventing the admission of patients who some believe do not require the conditions of maximum security of a Special Hospital. On the other hand some optimists believe that the number of patients in Special Hospitals can be substantially reduced. Special Hospital psychiatrists reply by pointing out that there will still be a need for Special Hospitals, particularly for those who are so dangerous that they could not be managed in regional units or who require more than a short stay. Many units have policies saying that patients will not be admitted if they are thought to require more than a year of treatment. Currently the average length of stay in Special Hospitals is about 5 years for Broadmoor and 9 for Rampton, and one of the main justifications for the existence of Special Hospitals is the range of occupational, educational and recreational facilities which is necessary for patients who are being deprived of their liberty for such long periods. As important as that are the moral considerations when one recognises that, according to the best information available, perhaps two out of three patients being detained in Special Hospitals would not re-offend if released.

Community forensic psychiatric facilities

Community forensic psychiatric facilities are only now being developed in the United Kingdom. The first community-based forensic psychiatric clinics were the Douglas Inch Centre in Glasgow which opened in 1964 (following the creation of the first post of consultant forensic psychiatrist some 10 years earlier) and the Portman Clinic in London which celebrated its Golden Jubilee in 1983.

Until only a few years ago the role of the consultant psychiatrist was limited to giving opinions for court proceedings on offenders in prison, and only rarely entailed conducting assessments or treatment in the community.

Literature on community forensic psychiatric facilities is sparse but Gunn (1971), using data from the Camberwell register which showed there were large numbers of patients requiring the help of a forensic psychiatrist, suggested there were many others who never received any form of psychiatric treatment and advocated specialised multi-disciplinary clinics to deal with acute psychosocial problems.

Craft (1974) described a community forensic psychiatric service in Wales dealing with 'a small difficult' group of patients who had committed sexual offences, property offences, offences of violence or arson. Craft found these mentally abnormal offenders could be successfully dealt with in an open and geographically isolated unit but stressed the need for more aftercare facilities and integration of male and female patients when dealing with large numbers of young male sexual offenders.

Bluglass (1977) described the work of the Midlands Centre for Forensic Psychiatry by an analysis of some 400 referrals to what was mainly an outpatient assessment and treatment service. About half the referrals came from magistrates' courts for assessment before sentence, with smaller numbers from the probation service, solicitors, general practitioners, other psychiatrists, prisons and juvenile and higher courts.

Another useful study on the development of secure facilities in NHS psychiatric hospitals was that of Carney and Nolan (1978). They described their unit as 'a crisis centre for the disturbed mentally ill', who were mainly psychotic patients exhibiting disturbed behaviour uncontrollable in ordinary wards. Many such units are in existence, though some hospitals (such as those in Oxford) still deny the need for any locked wards.

Invaluable information to assist the development of regional forensic psychiatric services was provided by Bowden (1977), whose paper outlined the number and distribution of forensic patients in the South East Thames Region. Commenting on the Butler Committee's recommendation that the guiding principle in the disposal of mentally abnormal offenders should be that they are admitted to the hospital best able to provide the treatment they need, Bowden refers to the views of others that disposal is influenced more by prejudice and lack of resources, as well as the attitude of nurses' unions.

Trade union activity has featured prominently in the development of forensic psychiatric services, resulting in the delay of the opening of one of the first interim secure units (Higgins, 1979). In February 1980 the failure of an NHS psychiatric hospital to admit a Broadmoor patient caused Lord Justice Brightman in the Court of Appeal to say: 'It is not a practical possibility in any well ordered organisation to have two independent decision-takers to exist side by side. The role of the nursing staff in decision-making on question of transfer is, in my view, a consultative role and not a decision-taking role.' Lord Justice Bridge added: 'nurses do not normally have any responsibility for decision-making, and they certainly, as far as I can see, do not have cast on them by the statute, either expressly or by necessary implication, any authority to take decisions of broad policy as to how the services of the hospital should be operated'. In 1983 the refusal of nursing staff to admit a patient who had been made the subject of a hospital order was condemned in the Appeal Court. (It may be noted here that the Health Secretary has never invoked his power to order an NHS hospital to admit on transfer a patient from a Special Hospital whereas the Home Secretary has not infrequently ordered hospitals to admit patients whose disposal is under the Criminal Procedure (Insanity) Act 1964.)

In an earlier paper Bowden (1975) showed a 40% reduction in beds in closed wards in South East Thames in the previous 5 years and argued that this, together with an increasing scarcity of common lodging house accommodation and the failure of the new psychiatric units in district general hospitals to admit difficult patients, resulted in a lack of facilities for mentally abnormal offenders. Bowden suggests that estimates of the need for secure unit provision have not taken account of those inappropriately placed patients.

Conclusions

Obviously the future of forensic psychiatry services depends on developments in the Special Hospitals, in secure units (both regional and 'interim'), in community services and in prisons, and the interplay between these sets of facilities.

Being at the end of the line as it were, the Special Hospitals are somewhat at the mercy of the other facilities, though they could clearly do more in terms of reaching out to them and demonstrating their willingness to co-operate more with flexible arrangements for interchange of patients according to their security needs. There have as yet been no scientifically respectable studies (other than that of Dell (1980) which is not directly relevant here) of patients in Special Hospitals who could be cared for in lesser degrees of security, though J. MacKeith and W. Spry in unpublished works suggest that large numbers could be handled in regional and local secure and non-secure facilities were they available.

Prisons seem almost to have given up their attempts to have mentally abnormal offenders (both serving sentence and on remand) admitted to NHS psychiatric hospitals and Special Hospitals. There appear to be serious problems in attracting high-quality staff to the Prison Medical

Service and morale has not been high, especially since well-publicised allegations of maltreatment of prisoners. As with Special Hospitals, much will depend on an increasing willingness by NHS hospitals to take patients from them. Consistent and constant reports of the number of mentally abnormal people in prison are too many to mention.

At the other end of the line from the Special Hospitals are the NHS community facilities; their development is likely to follow trends in care and financing in the NHS in general and psychiatry in particular. Serious concern has been expressed by psychiatrists and those representing patients and their families (e.g. the National Schizophrenia Fellowship) that the proposals to close mental hospitals will lead to more and more patients, many of them 'revolving door' petty offenders, being denied the treatment and asylum they need. Much hope therefore rests on the development of regional secure facilities, but there is still the fear that they will turn out to be a Pandora's Box. All will depend on their admission policies.

In their statement *Secure Facilities for Psychiatric Patients: A Comprehensive Policy* the Royal College of Psychiatrists (1980) said, in a section on which patients need increased security in hospitals or units other than Special Hospitals, that it was difficult to identify these patients:

> In general terms there is a group of patients who are not considered persistently dangerous but because of their unco-operative, periodic and often unpredictable behaviour many pose serious threats and dangers to themselves or to other people so that they cannot be managed in ordinary psychiatric hospitals or units. Some of these patients may be offenders, but many will not be. The criteria for their admission to a specialised unit should be seen in behavioural terms rather than rigidly depending upon psychiatric diagnosis or legal classification. Such patients would be those identified as creating continual difficulty in management and with a potential to respond to treatment facilities offered by special units; an essential element in determining suitability for admission.

The first criteria for admission to a secure unit were given by Faulk (1979), who said that the Knowle (Southampton) Unit's criteria after 2 years of operation included:

> (*a*) An agreement between the relevant doctors and staff that the patient is both mentally disordered and should be treated in hospital.
>
> (*b*) The patient's behaviour is too difficult or dangerous for him (or her) to be managed in an ordinary psychiatric ward, but is not

so difficult or dangerous that he/she requires the high security of a Special Hospital.

(c) The patient is either legally detained (e.g. by court order using the Mental Health Act) or is willing to stay as an 'informal' patient, or as a condition of probation.

Two years later Higgins (1981), on the basis of 4 years' experience running the Rainhill (Liverpool) Unit gave his criteria for admission as follows:

No absolute criteria for admission were set out when the ward opened, and none have emerged since. The following issues are currently considered important:

(1) All patients must present a physical danger to others, and as the ward is kept permanently locked all patients must be liable for detention under the Mental Health Act 1959.

(2) The level of physical security of the ward and the numbers of nursing staff available must be adequate for the management of the case.

(3) There must be an expectation that the patient will benefit from the regimen of the ward.

(4) The referring medical and nursing staff must agree to take a continuing interest in their patient and agree, subject to further consultation, to take him back when his behaviour has improved.

(5) If the patient is already in hospital it must be shown that he can no longer be managed in an open ward because (a) his behaviour has very seriously threatened the physical well-being of patients or staff and is likely to be repeated or (b) if less seriously threatening, his behaviour is so repetitive and disruptive that the ward regime is completely upset.

(6) Patients seen as outpatients are assessed as if they were already in hospital.

(7) A patient referred from a remand centre, prison or special hospital must have shown recent behaviour that would prevent him from being treated in an open ward or experience suggests that he requires longer-term management, more individual treatment, and closer supervision on discharge.

Most interim secure units have policies which state that patients with psychopathic disorder will not be admitted and only the Rainhill unit seems prepared to take other than short-stay patients: of their first 35 patients, 5 had a length of stay of 18 months or more and included one who had been there for 4 years and one for 3 years 2 months who was 'of expected long stay'.

Uncertainty about the criteria the DHSS uses in dealing with applications for admissions to Special Hospitals has been eased by MacCulloch (1982) and the position of the DHSS is further clarified in the *Memorandum on the Mental Health Act 1983* (Department of Health and Social Security, 1983) which says (para. 269):

> Special hospital admission is not generally considered suitable for patients who:
>
> (i) are suffering from severe mental impairment – unless there is a strong probability that the patient will seriously harm staff/other patients, if the opportunity presents;
>
> (ii) though exhibiting extreme disruptive or antisocial behaviour in the community or local hospital are unlikely to inflict serious physical injury;
>
> (iii) require close observation mainly to prevent self injury – unless this is associated with a probability of violence to others;
>
> (iv) require asylum/long term care but for whom lesser conditions of security would provide adequate protection for the public;
>
> (v) would simply benefit from the stability and support of a physically secure regime – unless they also present a risk of serious harm to the public at large;
>
> (vi) are under 16 years of age or over 60.
>
> Provision of comprehensive facilities for such patients is the responsibility of regional and district health authorities. Any lack of local provision for difficult to place patients will not usually be accepted as a reason for admission to a special hospital.

Whilst there is still some concern among Special Hospital psychiatrists that secure units will admit only short-stay patients and they will be left to handle the long-term patients, it is likely that these fears are ungrounded. There has been no let-up in the admission rate to Special Hospitals over the last few years and with the many mentally abnormal offenders still inappropriately placed it is sure to mean a constant demand for precious Special Hospital places. While Special Hospital placement may be initially desirable, the length of stay for most patients will depend not only on the willingness of secure units to take such patients but also on whether ordinary NHS psychiatric hospitals will accept patients without them having 'proved themselves' in regional secure units. Special Hospitals are attempting to combat this problem by changing their philosophy from one of 'removing dangerousness' (and leaving ordinary hospitals to complete treatment and rehabilitation) to developing their own rehabilitative procedures to make patients more able to cope with the ordinary hospital or community facilities when the time comes for them to leave the highly structured regimes of their institutions.

At the present time, however, bottlenecks have built up of patients waiting in Special Hospitals for places in secure units, and these facilities have so far made no impact on the number of mentally abnormal offenders in prisons. Doubts that regional secure units could solve the problem in the immediate future were raised by Parker and Tennent (1979) who described the fall in the number of hospital orders made over the years for admission to NHS hospitals and the corresponding burden placed on Special Hospitals and prisons. Parker and Tennent advocated better and more extensive psychiatric facilities within the penal system and evidently do believe secure units may be a Pandora's Box.

According to Brewer's *Dictionary of Phrase and Fable*, Pandora's Box is a present which seems valuable but which in reality is a curse; like that of Midas who found his food became gold, and therefore uneatable. When the Box was opened all the evils flew forth and have ever since continued to afflict the world. According to some accounts the last thing that flew out was Hope. Others say that Hope remained: let us hope so.

REFERENCES

Bluglass, R. (1977). Current developments in forensic psychiatry in the United Kingdom. *Psychiatric Journal of the University of Ottawa*, 11, 53–62.

Bowden, P. (1975). Liberty and psychiatry. *British Medical Journal*, iv, 94–6.

Bowden, P. (1977). The NHS practice of forensic psychiatry in one region. *Psychological Medicine*, 7, 141–8.

Carney, M.W.P. and Nolan, P.A. (1978). Area security unit in a psychiatric hospital. *British Medical Journal*, 1, 27–8.

Craft, M.J. (1974). A description of a new community forensic psychiatry service for doctors. *Medicine, Science and the Law*, 14, 268–72.

Dell, S. (1980). Transfer of Special Hospital patients to the NHS. *British Journal of Psychiatry*, 136, 222–34.

Department of Health and Social Security (1974). *Security in NHS Hospitals for the Mentally Ill and the Mentally Handicapped*. HMSO, London.

Department of Health and Social Security (1983). *Mental Health Act 1983. Memorandum on Parts I to VI, VIII and X*. HMSO, London.

Faulk, M. (1979). Mentally disordered offenders in an interim regional medium secure unit. *Criminal Law Review*, 686–95.

Gunn, J. (1971). Forensic psychiatry and psychopathic patients. *British Journal of Hospital Medicine*, 6, 260–4.

Hamilton, J.R. (1980). The development of Broadmoor 1863–1980. *Bulletin of the Royal College of Psychiatrists*, 4, 130–3.

Higgins, J. (1979). Rainford Ward, Rainhill Hospital. *Bulletin of the Royal College of Psychiatrists*, 3, 44–6.

Higgins, J. (1981). Four years' experience of an interim secure unit. *British Medical Journal*, 282, 889–93.

Home Office and Department of Health and Social Security (1974). *Interim Report of the Committee on Mentally Abnormal Offenders*. Cmnd 5698. HMSO, London.

Home Office and Department of Health and Social Security (1975). *Report of the Committee on Mentally Abnormal Offenders*. Cmnd 6244. HMSO, London.

MacCulloch, M. (1982). The Health Department's management of Special Hospital patients. In *Dangerousness: Psychiatric Assessment and Management*, ed. J.R. Hamilton and H. Freeman, pp. 101–5. Gaskell, London.

Ministry of Health (1961). *Special Hospitals. Report of Working Party*. HMSO, London.

Parker, E. and Tennent, G. (1979). The 1959 Mental Health Act and mentally abnormal offenders: a comparative study. *Medicine, Science and the Law*, 19, 29–38.

Patridge, R. (1953). *Broadmoor*. Chatto and Windus, London.

Royal College of Psychiatrists (1980). *Secure Facilities for Psychiatric Patients. A Comprehensive Policy*.

Royal College of Psychiatrists (1983). *The Future of the Special Hospitals*.

Snowden, P.R. (1985). *A Survey of the Regional Secure Unit Programme*. *British Journal of Psychiatry* (in press).

The role of psychiatry in prisons and 'the right to punishment'

JOHN GUNN

The legitimacy of psychiatry in prisons

Imprisonment may be such a stress that on occasions it can produce mental breakdown. Anybody who has worked in prisons, whether for criminals or for other detainees such as prisoners of war, will have seen examples of so-called prison psychosis, a paranoid delusional or hallucinatory state importing lots of prison paraphernalia into its content that tends to occur in personality disorders and remits when freedom is regained. Equally it is common to see severe, highly understandable depressions at the beginning of a long sentence, or at a point where an individual begins to comprehend the enormity of the events which led him to prison – perhaps a killing. The increased suicide rate in prisons, especially during the first few months of imprisonment, is probably related, in part, to depressions of this kind.

Some would say that not only do prisons generate psychiatric problems but they also collect them inappropriately and act as unofficial mental hospitals for individuals who should be in health care. A mental health census within the English prison system has estimated that approximately one third of sentenced men could be regarded as psychiatric cases (Gunn et al., 1978). This is not to suggest that all these men required inpatient care. The majority were suffering from personality disorders, chronic neuroses, alcoholism, and drug dependency. Nevertheless 20% had previously been patients in the National Health Service (NHS) and many showed severe anxiety and depression; perhaps 1% were psychotic.

If British prisons really do take an excessive number of mentally disordered people, perhaps this is because there is a special relationship between crime and mental disorder. Stated thus the hypothesis is too simplistic to be evaluated. What can be said is that while there are no special relationships between mental disorder and common offences such as motoring crimes or theft, there are *some* special relationships between mental disorder and behaviour – for example between alcohol abuse and assault, between disturbed sexuality and sexual offences. It is also true that patients with chronic intractable disorders such as schizophrenia, chronic mania, mental handicap or severe personality disorder are more likely than healthy people to behave badly and land up in the criminal justice system. It is these chronic patients that create disputes between services. Nobody wants them. Doctors and nurses will bend over backwards to define them as normal or to fill their facilities so that they do not have to accept them as patients. Courts see them as a stage army costing a great deal of money, clearly not responding to a neat model of deterrence, and therefore in need of treatment to cure them. Prison authorities despair because the gaols ultimately find themselves saddled with these individuals. Like everybody else the prisons have no cures to offer, but worse they find themselves in an ethical dilemma because their disciplinary system of management is ineffective for many in this category. It is probably the tendency to reject these patients which led Dr Orr, when he was Director of the Prison Medical Service, to say that 'mentally abnormal offenders are entering prisons . . . because hospital places are not forthcoming . . . Hospitals have clearly sought to divest themselves of their traditional role of providing asylum for people unable to cope elsewhere' (Orr, 1978).

Does all this add up to a legitimate role for the psychiatrist in the prison? Probably, but it is not really the reason that he is there. In the eighteenth century doctors began to take an interest in prisons because of infections, especially typhus (so-called gaol fever). In the middle of the nineteenth century there developed an interest in removing from the penal system the more obviously mentally deranged. It was at that point that the diagnosis of insanity became one of the concerns of the prison doctor. So one of the basic drives for prison psychiatry was the traditional one of protecting the insane from the full rigours of the law. By no means all of the mentally disordered could be removed from the prisons and so, as early as 1850, special facilities were set aside for them. One of the hulks in the Thames was designated as an 'invalid depot' for both physically and mentally infirm and by 1855 the medical officer there had 100 'weak minded' convicts in his care. By 1889 a Home Office circular was urging magistrates not to sentence insane persons to imprisonment but to commit them to an asylum instead. At the beginning of this century Parkhurst was the prison for those 'unfit for ordinary penal discipline because of some mental disability'.

Grendon prison

An historical analysis of prison psychiatry, which has been documented elsewhere (Gunn *et al.*, 1978), suggests that the predominant philosophy of the Home Office has been to clear as many mentally disordered people as possible from the prisons, but this has failed in the face of resistance from health care systems which have the right of refusal. There was just one period of doubt about the wisdom of this philosophy and that was when the notion of treating crime by medical and psychological techniques became fashionable, the period of so-called positivism. This period led to the famous East–Hubert Report of 1939 and eventually to Grendon prison. The report actually said that 'the main object of psychotherapy in criminal work is to prevent crime being committed and repeated by the individual'.

Some years ago several of us had a close look at Grendon prison. By the time Grendon had opened in 1962 it was designed as a therapeutic community modelled on Henderson Hospital and the war-time group treatment at Northfield Hospital. It was taking neurotic and personality-disordered men who were mainly well-established recidivists in their middle twenties. On average they were serving quite long sentences ($3\frac{1}{2}$ years) and had a lot of previous prison experience (3 years). They were subjected to an intensive therapeutic atmosphere based on groups, democracy as far as is possible within a prison, and a remarkable equality between prisoners and officers. We found that this prison was indisputably different from all other prisons in atmosphere; indeed it was the model on which the special unit at Barlinnie was based. It was clearly able to manage violent men and sex offenders that other prisons could not manage. It improved prisoners' attitudes to authority figures, it gave them more social self-confidence and it markedly reduced the prisoner's neurotic symptomatology. However, the prison was no better or worse than any other in influencing the post-release reconviction rate of its inmates. In other words it turned out that Grendon, a psychiatric prison, was good at psychiatry and indeed at management of prisoners but made little difference to reconviction rates. True we suggested that some improvement in reconviction rates might be effected by proper Grendon aftercare, which at present does not exist, but the prison as currently established does not cure people of crime. Such a finding which would probably have surprised East and Hubert, unexpectedly still surprises people today. Most of the skills employed in the prison, whilst having their roots in psychology, could in fact be, indeed are, learned by ordinary prison staff and the level of medical involvement required is mainly supervisory.

Remands for reports

British prisons are centres for the psychiatric assessments of prisoners for the courts. In many countries if a court wants to know about the mental state of an accused at the time of an alleged offence it will send him to a psychiatric hospital for a psychiatric assessment. Not so in Britain. If he needs custody he will be sent to a remand prison and be examined by a prison doctor. In an average year the prison medical service provides over 170 such reports a week, or nearly 9000 over the year. True, many of the accused men will also be examined by a psychiatrist of their own choosing, but that examination will also be carried out within the prison. Given the reluctance of hospitals and NHS psychiatrists to get involved in work with offenders this may seem a perfectly reasonable way of doing things. However, it has a number of important disadvantages.

Most obviously it is sending untried and sometimes entirely innocent people to prison simply to get a medical report; a clear injustice. On occasions people charged with offences that do not carry a sentence of imprisonment are remanded in custody simply in order for the court to have a medical report; another injustice. Next it removes all pressure from the NHS to provide proper assessment facilities. Fourthly, assessments in prison cannot be as full and as relevant as they would be in a good hospital setting: the prison environment is a highly abnormal one in which to look for signs and symptoms of an individual's possible illness; special investigations are difficult to obtain; opinions from other specialists such as psychologists, occupational therapists and so on are in very short supply; therapeutic trials with anything but drugs are virtually impossible; and contact with relatives is distorted by the prison context. Lastly and very importantly, assessments in prison bias medical reports to prison disposals. Any doctor will discuss and recommend facilities, treatments, arrangements with which he is familiar. Prison doctors are no exception; they will think first and foremost of the arrangements available within the prisons such as psychotherapy, therapeutic communities, physical treatments and the like and recommend these to the courts. Even if they are convinced that hospital care is required within the NHS or a Special Hospital all they can do is try and persuade a doctor from an appropriate centre to visit and hope that he sees sufficient pathology on the day he attends to make him agree.

Gibbens and his colleagues (Gibbens, Soothill and Pope, 1977) have shown that this pattern of remanding offenders in custody to obtain a medical report is much more marked in London than in small towns, but it does occur everywhere. Bail hostels and indeed bail clinics have been set up in an attempt to reduce the numbers of individuals remanded in custody for medical reports but they have had only a minimal effect. The Mental Health Act 1983 also attempts to reduce the numbers and produce a swing towards assessments in hospital by means of two new provisions: remands to hospital and interim hospital orders. However, it is difficult to see how such legislation will make much difference when the real problems are resources and attitudes. It has always been possible to ask for an offender to be remanded on bail with a condition of residence in hospital.

When Dr Paul Bowden examined the men going through Brixton prison in order to obtain medical reports (Bowden, 1978*a*) he found that those who received a recommendation for treatment tended to have a diagnosis of acute mental illness and had in the past been admitted more frequently to mental hospitals; they were assessed as difficult to manage, sometimes threatening and potentially violent. Those who were not recommended for treatment more often had a history of excessive drinking and they had more extensive criminal histories. Some 14 months later nearly three quarters of the men who went to hospital had been discharged (Bowden, 1978*b*). Those sent to hospital fell into three groups: men with acute psychoses for whom treatment was definitely beneficial, men who remained behaviourally disturbed in spite of improvements in their mental states, and a group with chronic disorders for whom admission was not beneficial. The two groups with improved mental states represented only 5% of the initial receptions to Brixton prison.

This peculiarity of the British prison system is then, to say the least, highly inefficient. The process of remand for a medical report is probably inefficient whether the remand is to prison or to hospital. The inefficiency may even be a virtue for it means that strenuous efforts are being made to avoid missing a treatable case. What is not a virtue is the endangering of justice which the British system produces when it locks up large numbers of accused people – some of whom are innocent, some of whom are not going to receive prison sentences, some of whom are not even eligible for prison sentences – simply in order to get a medical opinion which is often biased towards prison care.

Of course even systems which remand people to hospital carry some of the same dangers. In the United States the courts have the power to remand people to hospital for reports and frequently do so, but the hospitals are sometimes as tough and prison-like as English gaols and the health care terminology may therefore not impress the offender very much. However, when the onus is on the health care system it is easier to improve efficiency and justice and get a more therapeutic system. In some parts of the United States outpatient services called community forensic

clinics are being set up and courts are being encouraged to refer to them
for opinions rather than to the state hospitals. Beran and Toomey (1979)
have studied such a development in Ohio and shown that the service not
only costs less but also leads to more outpatient and straightforward
psychiatric recommendations than did the old system which put a heavy
emphasis on incarceration in Lima State Hospital. At the conclusion of
their study Gibbens *et al.* (1977) ask us not to concentrate the practice of
forensic psychiatry in the hands of a few people. They believe that the best
hope of integrating the mentally abnormal offender into the community is
to treat him as far as possible as an ordinary patient; this will overcome the
tendency to regard him (and for him to regard himself) as an outcast or as a
special case. They urge that the majority of offenders with psychiatric
problems should be dealt with by general psychiatrists or by generalists
with a special interest.

Interim conclusion

So, for those who become mentally sick as a result of imprisonment and for those who are sick and dumped into prisons by social
pressures there can surely be no question in a caring society that there is a
role for the psychiatrist in prison. Equally, as long as courts and hospitals
put mentally sick people into prison on remand then it can be argued that
an assessment role for the psychiatrist will always be there. The difficulty
of this position is that the presence of the psychiatrist within the prison
system may actually encourage society and its courts to divert more
mentally abnormal people to prison. For this reason psychiatrists should
not participate in prison work on the mistaken assumption that crime can
be cured by medical, psychological, or quasi-medical techniques, but only
on the clear ethical basis that wherever there are sick people, the medical
profession should attend with skill.

The right to punishment

Several reviews have demonstrated that reconviction rates seem
unaffected by prison regimes (e.g. Brody, 1976). The right-to-punish-
ment lobby is saying 'Why not simply forget about treatment – which
tends to be longer and more intrusive than punishment – and simply dole
out the appropriate dose of punishment, appropriate that is, in terms of
the going rate for the crime committed?' The concept of a right to
punishment is also partly a reaction against the paternalism of psychiatry.
It says 'Who are these self-appointed saviours of my soul? Why should I
be made better? I know what the risks of crime are; I can take the
punishment when I slip up.' It is partly a reaction to the horror of what

some civil rights groups call the psycho-cop. That is it is a reaction against the notion that psychiatrists should be able to extend sentences indefinitely on a flimsy predictive basis when they consider some captive or patient to be dangerous. It is partly a reaction against the tendency to label antisocial behaviour as mad and thus devalue what may be in the eyes of the perpetrator a perfectly rational or legitimate act. An extreme example of this is the locking up of political dissidents in Russia as mad on the basis that anybody who holds the view they do about their country must be mad.

In 1973 a young girl was sitting alone in a railway carriage; in jumped a young man. When the train was between stations he jumped up, opened his trousers, advanced towards the girl and demanded that she kiss him. When she refused he squeezed her round the neck till she passed out. After she recovered from this he forced his penis into her mouth. A man already attending hospital for sexual problems who had recently been admitted as an inpatient was arrested for the crimes. He protested his innocence but was identified by the girl on an identification parade and he was convicted. For 10 years he has continued to protest his innocence and has adduced quite a lot of evidence to support his alibi, which has convinced a number of eminent lawyers and a lot of television viewers. That, however, is beside the point. He was found guilty on a majority verdict and sentenced to 4 years in prison. Thirty-two months later he was due to be released but he was not released. Just before his prison sentence was due to expire he was transferred to a Special Hospital. Nobody has ever suggested that he was mentally ill. He was regarded as a dangerous, incurable psychopath who may attack young women again and possibly kill them. He appealed to Mental Health Review Tribunals but they took his doctors' advice and continued his detention (Young and Hill, 1983). Not surprisingly he is angry and believes that psychiatry has dealt him a much harsher sentence than did the penal system. He wanted the right to be treated as a criminal, to be punished and then allowed to be free rather than to be regarded as a patient with a chronic disorder requiring continuous restraint. Who can blame him?

Psychiatrists cannot ignore public interests and public safety. To put it at its mildest it is not in the patient's best interests to be allowed to assault, rape, or kill someone and the psychiatric profession would soon be in disrepute if it argued otherwise. More than that the public does expect the psychiatrist to protect them from dangerously insane people and will always employ 'experts' to give advice about these issues. If doctors refuse to give such advice then others will step forward instead. However, there is no reason to suppose that the only way of dealing with these questions is in the way outlined above. There must be justice and methods of appeal even in medical matters (e.g. Floud and Young, 1981; Gunn, 1982). In the case described the doctors and the tribunals may have been right; maybe the patient was highly dangerous, requiring long-term incarceration. However, it seems manifestly unfair to single out a man for long-term protective custody without explaining, in open court, why he is getting such a heavy sentence and without giving him the opportunity, again in open court, of arguing with the facts presented and putting a different point of view. It also seems unfair to impose protective custody on him, without warning, at the end of a valid tariff sentence imposed by a court. He should have known from the beginning what his fate was to be.

Some attempt to deal with the injustices mentioned above has been made in the Mental Health Act 1983; in particular a psychopath is no longer detainable unless he is regarded as treatable. What treatability means is anybody's guess, but it is to be hoped that in future there will be no danger of using any Special or other hospitals purely for protective custody in the case of psychopaths, and that at the regular Mental Health Review Tribunals questions will be asked about progress as well as about dangerousness. A further safeguard in the new Act is that all patients, even those on restriction orders, will have access to Mental Health Review Tribunals with real powers. What advantage, if any, this brings remains to be seen. There is no evidence that the Home Office is less fair or less well informed in its decision-making about the release of patients than the average Mental Health Review Tribunal. The reverse is likely to be the case.

Restriction orders

There are two minor changes which would do a lot to remove from Britain the strange plea for the right to be punished, and which are within our grasp without changes in legislation. The first would be for judges to make more use of the timed restriction order. Restriction orders are orders imposed by judges after a person has been convicted and a hospital order has been made. In effect they remove the power of discharging the patient from the doctor and give it to the Home Secretary. Such restriction orders can be for a limited period or without limit of time, in which event they have the same force as a life sentence as far as discharge and licensing is concerned. The vast majority of restriction orders are without limit of time because, understandably, the witnesses and the court do not want to guess when the patient will no longer be dangerous. Further, such orders are often made in respect of someone who would have attracted a life sentence anyway; someone, say, who has killed. However there are occasions when an accused is found guilty of a lesser offence, say an assault, an arson, or a burglary, which would have attracted a fixed sentence of, say, 5 to 10 years. Instead, he is diverted to hospital because of a medical condition, perhaps depression or schizophrenia. In these cases it would seem much more just to impose the restriction order in accordance with the tariff for the crime committed and allow the medical questions to be considered separately. So if, say, a depressed man starts a fire he would receive a hospital order and a restriction order for a period appropriate for arson, say 7 years. If he is ready for discharge before the 7 years is up then the usual dialogue between doctor and Home Office takes place. If he remains unwell for more than 7 years then the decision reverts to the medical officer alone after the restriction order has ended. In this way patients would not appear to receive longer penal sentences than their healthy counterparts.

Parole

The second minor reform would be for psychiatrists to eschew considering dangerousness and release issues in a case unless it is clear that there are definite psychiatric factors. Currently, for example, psychiatrists are involved in *all* parole decisions whether or not the prisoners are mentally normal. It would help to answer the jibe 'psycho-cop' if it could be claimed with confidence that psychiatrists are never involved in non-psychiatric penal decisions.

Conclusion

It seems, then, that whilst a great deal of good psychiatric work is done within our overstretched prisons, they are being used for the wrong purpose when they are used as substitute mental hospitals. In particular psychiatric assessment should be carried out in hospitals which are fully equipped for this purpose, and this means all hospitals, Special, medium secure, and open. Prison psychiatrists are severely under-resourced and they need a lot more support from their NHS colleagues. These days they do not have time to believe that they are offering medical cures for crime; they are too busy with basic psychiatry, which would be better tackled elsewhere.

To finally lay to rest the right to punishment issue we should do a number of straightforward things. Firstly we should ensure that mentally abnormal offenders are welcome within the NHS. Then we should ensure that hospitals are not used expediently to tackle problems which courts cannot face openly, in particular that they are not used simply as places of protective custody. Thirdly we should redirect the interests of general psychiatry to the care of the chronic patient so that individuals with long-standing personality disorders and other intractable problems can genuinely regard the doctor as the caring agency who is actually on his side. Lawyers, social workers, nurses, doctors, can all be helpful to patients with schizophrenia, chronic mania, antisocial personality disorder, alcoholism, and the like; however, the one who is going to have the greatest impact in the long run is the one who is actually there. We should encourage courts and penal administrators to separate health and penal matters more clearly, and psychiatrists should ensure that they do not get involved with the sentencing and release of normal offenders.

REFERENCES

Beran, N.J. and Toomey, B.G. (1979). *Mentally Ill Offenders and the Criminal Justice System.* Praeger, New York.

Bowden, P. (1978*a*). Men remanded into custody for medical reports: the selection for treatment. *British Journal of Psychiatry*, 133, 320–31.

Bowden, P. (1978*b*). Men remanded into custody for medical reports: the outcome of the treatment recommendation. *British Journal of Psychiatry*, 133, 323–8.

Brody, S.R. (1976). *The Effectiveness of Sentencing: A Review of the Literature.* Home Office Research Study No. 35. HMSO, London.

East, W.M. and Hubert, W.H. de B. (1939). *The Psychological Treatment of Crime.* HMSO, London.

Floud, J. and Young, W. (1981). *Dangerousness and Criminal Justice.* Heinemann, London.

Gibbens, T.C.N., Soothill, K.L. and Pope, P.J. (1977). *Medical Remands in the Criminal Court.* Oxford University Press, Oxford.

Gunn, J. (1982). An English psychiatrist looks at dangerousness. *Bulletin of the American Academy of Psychiatry and the Law*, 10, 143–53.

Gunn, J., Robertson, G.R., Dell, S. and Way, C. (1978). *Psychiatric Aspects of Imprisonment.* Academic Press, London.

Orr, J.H. (1978). The imprisonment of mentally disordered offenders. *British Journal of Psychiatry*, 133, 194–9.

Young, M. and Hill, P. (1983). *Rough Justice.* BBC, London.

Human rights in mental health

LARRY GOSTIN

Some years ago there was an action brought against a medical man for allegedly signing an order for the detention of a patient, and since then a great many medical men have refused to sign orders for admission into an asylum. It appears to me that there should be some relief to medical men . . . that you must prove malice before you can punish for any action of that sort.
(Sir Trevor Lawrence, 1877)

The opinion of any medical practitioner shall not be admissible as evidence of the insanity of a person.
(An amendment tabled to the Lunacy Regulations Bill 1845 by Montague Smith, MP)

The relativistic nature of human rights in mental health

Both lawyers and psychiatrists have traditionally presumed that their approach to mental health is in the person's interests (Gostin, 1983*a*, *b*). In any discussion of the 'human rights' of mentally disordered people it is important to examine the term. A human right is no more than an entitlement due – legally or morally – to a human being. If we construe the term to mean a statutory right, it takes us no further, for it is one which government can choose whether or not to legislate for a particular group. A statutory right has no constancy and will deviate over time and across national boundaries. To most of us a human right suggests some permanence: for example, the right not to use medicine for political purposes. But even this human right presupposes a moral choice between two opposing objectives, i.e. restricting the practice of medicine for the benefit of the individual is more important than using the medical profession to achieve political or social objectives. The moral choice is not as clear in other mental health matters for much depends upon what individual interest is intended to be protected: a person's health and wellbeing, or his self-determination and liberty. The human right would be framed quite differently depending upon the value chosen. In the former case emphasis would be placed upon facilitating access to care without legal encumbrance. (This assumes that treatment and care are always beneficial and that there should be no encumbrance.) In the latter case, the usual legal controls – both substantive and procedural – against unjustified confinement or coercion would be guaranteed. (It is sometimes wrongly assumed that legal safeguards are, by their nature, anti-therapeutic; and that lawyers by their actions are critical of psychiatry.)

There probably exists no ideal moral conduct in mental health; nor would any solution merit universal moral approval. The humanistic value I will pursue is to maximise a person's choice as to where his own interests lie. Where society is to withdraw that basic human prerogative because it claims the individual is incapable of rationally exercising choice, it must give the person the opportunity to refute that proposition before an impartial decision-maker. Indeed, where human rights judgments have been made, not on the basis of statute, but grounded upon superior constitutional guarantees, the right to be protected almost invariably relates to the procedural right of due process.

Judicial review of compulsory admission

The 'due process' principle is founded upon the general right to a determination by a court of law concerning the need for deprivation of liberty or self-determination. This principle is to be found in the International Covenant of Civil and Political Rights (Totsuka, 1983), the European Convention of Human Rights (Gostin, 1982) and in national constitutions such as that of the United States (Herr, Arons and Wallace, 1983). In each case the general right has applied in respect of mentally disordered people to establish the principle that, save for short-term admission as a crisis-intervention measure, there must be judicial review of compulsory admission to hospital.

The concept of judicial review has been closely associated with a legalistic approach to mental health. Judicial approval of the admissions decision has been criticised as attaching a criminal veneer to the mentally disordered and, more importantly, imposing technical procedural barriers to access to needed care. Intervention by a court can appear senseless if its purpose is to obtain the 'right' decision. There is no reason to presume that courts make 'better' decisions than doctors in respect of the exercise of compulsory powers of admission, any more than criminal courts can decipher guilt or innocence more accurately than the prosecutor or police. I use this analogy intentionally because the human rights guarantee under question – i.e. judicial review of confinement – is the same in both cases; and in both cases the justification for judicial review is not obtaining the 'correct' result but ensuring fairness to the individual concerned.

The purpose of judicial review in both contexts is neither truth nor expediency; although we like to think that the judicial process will provide the decision-maker with fuller information, thus assisting in obtaining a just or more accurate result. (Although there is no evidence that this is so.) The purpose of a court review is to give the individual, faced with the consequence of the drastic diminution in personal autonomy, the right of access to an independent decision-maker who will consider all the evidence which the individual can bring to bear to refute the case for the deprivation of autonomy. It is not too much to require of a society to compel it to allow the individual the opportunity of a dispassionate review to establish clearly that there is a justification for interference with a person's ordinary freedom. Further, the fact that the intended objective is 'treatment', not 'punishment', does not obscure the fact that what is at stake is a person's liberty.

Recognition of this fundamental principle does not require us to take the analogy with the criminal trial too far by requiring identical procedural safeguards. The intention behind judicial review in the mental health context is a full and fair hearing without secrecy. This requires basic procedural fairness including the right to appear with publicly funded representation and independent expert advice; to have knowledge of all of the information available to the court and to be able to comment on and question evidence and witnesses; and to be given reasons for the court's decision. Other formal criminal due process procedures such as a jury trial, criminal standard of proof, the right to remain silent and the demonstration of past criminal behavior do not serve any major objectives in the mental health context. Informality of atmosphere, as with a multi-disciplinary tribunal in England and Wales, can avoid many of the objections to judicial review.

The charge that judicial review, other than in emergency cases, impedes access to treatment is ill-founded. It presumes that which still has to be impartially established, i.e. that the person requires treatment which can most effectively be given in hospital. It may be that introduction of legal procedures dissuades mental health professionals from treating those who, in their opinion, require it. But it is not the procedure which prevents treatment, but the professional's aversion to the procedure. It is right that, if society gives a professional group the authority to exercise a compulsory power affecting the freedom of the individual, it should lay down criteria and procedures for the exercise of that power; and that an established judicial process will be used to determine the social questions involved. We should have a reasonable expectation that those charged with responsibility will not be dissuaded by the necessity of judicial review for the purpose of confirming the professional's judgment; medical judgment, as with any other professional judgment, can be fallible.

Consent to treatment

The question often arises whether, having judicially determined the need for compulsory admission, there is the need for further review of decisions to exercise certain compulsory powers such as treatment. Much depends upon whether the initial judicial determination sought to determine whether the person is capable of exercising the right in question. Ideally a court reviewing a decision to compulsorily admit a patient would seek to determine whether he was capable of refusing treatment. Most statutes do not specify criteria which would enable courts to do this. However, even if they did the task might well prove formidable. The question of whether a person is competent to refuse treatment varies over time and according to the treatment involved. It is increasingly recognised that not all compulsorily detained patients are incapable of understanding the nature and purpose of particular treatments. A psychotically jealous husband, for example, may pose a real threat to his wife, and may be properly detained. He may, however, understand the purpose of the medication being administered and be aware of its adverse effects (it may make him drowsy or cause him to shake or lose concentration).

The foundation of the common law right to impose treatment rests upon the presumed incompetency of the patient to consent. There is no justification for removal of a person's right to self-determination unless specific incompetency can be proved, i.e. the person is incapable of exercising the particular judgment in question for himself. In other branches of medicine it is accepted that a competent person can choose to refuse what is good for him even if it causes anguish or death. There is no reason to alter this doctrine for the psychiatric patient who is able to exercise rational choice (Gostin, 1981).

Peer review

The question then arises as to who determines whether the patient has competency. From the patient's perspective there is a disagreement between himself and his doctor as to where his best interests lie. For one of the parties to that relationship to determine (because the patient does not agree with him or for other reasons) that the patient is incompetent will not be regarded as fair and effective decision-making. For the patient to see the resolution of that disagreement as being fair he has to be able to present his perspective to a dispassionate decision-maker in whom he has confidence. Neither the patient nor the public would have confidence in peer review. Professional self-regulation is always suscep-tible to the criticism that it is not sufficiently dispassionate, energetic and open. This is not intended as a criticism of the medical profession, but would be an accepted principle of fairness in reviewing decisions of any professional group.

The question of whether a treatment is beneficial is solely a medical/scientific decision. However, whether that treatment should be imposed upon the individual through force of law is not exclusively a clinical question but a social/lay judgment. The question is not what is good for the patient, but whether he can make a choice within broad boundaries of reasonableness – whether his ability to exercise choice is so defective that society deems it necessary to impose a specific course of action on him.

No single solution can warrant being called a human rights imperative. Yet, in this context a lay review – allowing the patient to present evidence, to know the reasons why treatment is thought necessary and to comment upon those reasons – best effectuates a person's rights. From the patient's perspective there is no human rights principle more fundamental than to give him access to a decision-making process which he can have confidence in. This requires, as in any other related context, that the patient can present his personal perspective and evidence fully and fairly, and that the decision-maker can be regarded as fully independent, and not representative of any professional point of view.

Entitlement to services

The entitlement of mentally disordered people to appropriate services has never found definitive expression as a human right. The ostensible justification for this is that there is no absolute level of resources and treatment which could be used across national boundaries. Moreover, access to services has traditionally been a prerogative given by government through statute and not through constitutional guarantee (International Commission of Jurists, 1981). Yet, a principle of equality within national boundaries could be fashioned to state a cogent argument for an entitlement to services – i.e. services not based upon charitable or professional discretion, but upon enforceable rights. The rules of equity and fairness are deeply entrenched principles of constitutional law. From a broad legal perspective, a government is not obliged to provide health and social services. However, once it chooses to provide services it cannot arbitrarily exclude certain individuals or client groups. If there is an unreasonable denial of a service, the remedy is, or should be, provided by law.

In the United States the right to treatment or habilitation has been put forward as a duty which logically must flow from the exercise of compulsory powers of detention. The *sine qua non* of therapeutic detention is the patient's need for treatment. The absence of minimal treatment removes the justification for detention. The United States Supreme Court has gone as far as saying that the compulsory detention of a *non-dangerous* patient without treatment is unconstitutional. It has not, however, enunciated a general right to treatment or habilitation (*O'Connor v. Donaldson*, 1975).

The European Commission of Human Rights has used Article 3 of the Convention of Human Rights to seek to compel minimal standards of care (*A. v. United Kingdom*, 1980; Gostin, 1983*a*). Article 3, which prohibits inhuman and degrading treatment, has been used to seek to establish the right to treatment, but the Commission has never gone this far. The dissenting opinion of Mr Opsahl ably summarises the position of the Commission (*B. v. United Kingdom*, 1981):

> All members seem to be agreed that the case had a number of aspects causing concern under Article 3. There is no need to go over details again: the facts of overcrowding and poor facilities in the institution were disturbing, the doubts as to the merits of the decisions to place and keep the applicant there were considerable, and the difficulties in achieving the purported objective of treatment were obvious. The question is whether any of this, separately or all of it added together, can amount to failure to observe the standards required by Article 3.

The Commission found no violation of Article 3, arguing that each of the above elements of harm should be viewed in the disjunctive; the Commission also did not take account of proportionality between the seriousness of the original offence and the subsequent harm. Mr Opsahl concludes: 'The part about proportionality is rejected . . . on the formal ground that the consequences were not a part of a "penalty" but of a "treatment"; an argument I fail to understand since Article 3 prohibits certain "treatment" as well as punishment.'

The Commission's decision that no violation of Article 3 occurred was narrow (eight votes to five), and did not entirely close the door to a future judgment of violation based upon serious harm and neglect. Yet, this does not indicate any likelihood that the Commission will find any general right to treatment.

Conclusion

There has been considerable recent international concern about the human rights of mental patients. The persistent criticism of the use of psychiatry for political purposes is a proper, but predictable response of western society. Yet the suggestion that admission to hospital and treatment genuinely intended for therapeutic purposes may violate minimal standards of human dignity and autonomy is a new departure in the international human rights field. The movement for the legal rights of patients began in North America in the 1960s primarily by judicial action. By 1978 the World Health Organisation had published a comparative survey of mental health legislation (Curran and Harding, 1978). Already a series of cases against the United Kingdom had been filed with the European Commission of Human Rights, and by 1981 the lead case had been successful (*X* v. *United Kingdom*). The International Commission of Jurists (1980) formed two working parties at the invitation of the United Nations to draft a set of principles for the protection of persons of unsound mind. Both working parties accepted the US and European position of the right of judicial review. However, the relativistic nature of human rights in mental health can be illustrated by the fact that the two working parties took irreconcilable positions on certain key features of the Declaration, including the concept of treatability. A final document is now in the ratification process at the United Nations; a similar document has also been published by the Council of Europe (1983).

The absence of any general right to treatment continues to present the greatest dilemma for psychiatry and law. It is ironic that a human right can be fashioned from the concept of freedom from treatment, but that access to adequate treatment and care cannot. However, individual governments can create the right to services which is enforceable at the behest of the individual. This has been done in the United States with the Developmental Disabilities Legislation and in England and Wales with the aftercare Section in the Mental Health Act 1983 (Gostin, 1985). Creating an entitlement to services through statute is one of the most positive recent changes in the legal approach to mental health, which I have referred to elsewhere as 'the ideology of entitlement' (Gostin, 1983*a*). The joining together of psychiatrists and lawyers for this purpose can offer an effective common strategy and point of agreement for the future.

REFERENCES

Books, articles and international declarations
Council of Europe (1983). Recommendation No. R(83)2 of the Committee of Ministers to Member States Concerning the Legal Protection of Persons Suffering from Mental Disorder Placed as Involuntary Patients. Adopted by the Committee of Ministers on 22 February 1983 at the 356th Meeting of the Ministers' Deputies.

Curran, W.J. and Harding, T. (1978). *The Law and Mental Health: Harmonizing Objectives.* World Health Organisation, Geneva.

Gostin, L. (1981). Observations on consent to treatment and review of clinical judgment in psychiatry: a discussion paper. *Journal of the Royal Society of Medicine*, 74, 742–52.

Gostin, L. (1982). Human rights, judicial review and the mentally disordered offender. *Criminal Law Review* (1982), 779–93.

Gostin, L. (1983*a*). The ideology of entitlement: the application of contemporary legal approaches to psychiatry. In *Mental Illness: Changes and Trends*, ed. P. Bean, pp. 27–54. Wiley, Chichester.

Gostin, L. (1983*b*). Contemporary social historical perspectives on mental health reform. *Journal of Law and Society*, 10, 47–69.

Gostin, L. (1985). *Mental Health Services and the Law*, Shaw and Sons, London.

Herr, S., Arons, S. and Wallace, R. (1983). *Legal Rights and Mental Health Care.* Lexington, Mass.

International Commission of Jurists and International Association of Penal Law (1981). *The Protection of Persons of Unsound Mind.* International Association of Penal Law, Siracusa, Sicily.

Lawrence, T. (1877). Evidence to Select Committee to Inquire into the Operations of the Lunacy Act as Regards the Security Afforded against Violations of Personal Liberty, 12 February 1877, para. 4839.

Totsuka, E. (1983). Mental health and human rights under the International Covenant on Civil and Political Rights. In *Proceedings of the International Congress on Psychiatry, Law and Ethics*, ed. J. Carmi. (In press.)

Cases

X v. *United Kingdom*, application number 6998/75. Judgment of the European Court of Human Rights, 5 November 1981.

B v. *United Kingdom*, application number 6870/75. Report of the European Commission of Human Rights, 7 October 1981.

A v. *United Kingdom*, application number 6840/74. Report of the European Commission of Human Rights, 16 July 1980.

O'Connor v. *Donaldson*, 422 US 563 (1975).

Changes in mental health legislation as indicators of changing values and policies

MARGARET A. SOMERVILLE

Change raises mixed emotions. In particular, fear associated with the unknown and doubt caused by change, are especially likely to occur when trans-disciplinary activity takes place, as it does in law's involvement in psychiatry.[1] In fact, this activity and the change that it generates may even be perceived as a crisis by some psychiatrists. The Chinese write the word 'crisis' by combining the symbols for two other words. Those words are 'danger' and 'opportunity'. Both factors are present at this critical time of transition from the old to the new mental health law in England and in other countries where similar changes have taken place.

The aim in the first part of this paper is to identify some of the major changes which have been enacted in the new English legislation and then, by way of comparison with the old legislation and with the approaches adopted in other jurisdictions, particularly the Canadian jurisdiction of Ontario, to try to articulate the shifts in values and policies represented by these new laws. This is not an easy task and, in itself, involves value judgment. In fact, the questions asked, the values detected, the range of values used as a base-line, and the relative importance the values are given, all involve elements of value judgment. However, some measure of objectivity is possible. In particular, one result of identifying and articulating underlying principles is that these principles can be judged, not only by the person carrying out that task, but also by others and, often, somewhat more objectively.

In the second part of the paper, more general value and policy considerations relevant to the structure established by mental health legislation will be addressed. In the third part, some of the pillars of this

The references to the English Mental Health Act in this paper are mainly to the Mental Health (Amendment) Act. Since the paper was written the Mental Health (Amendment) Act and the Mental Health Act 1959 have been consolidated into the Mental Health Act 1983 for England and Wales.

structure will be examined. These include the role of law in relation to medicine, the nature of professions and how they are regulated, and principles related to decision-making.

The relationship between the first and latter parts of this paper and the difference between them, in terms of the approach taken, can be articulated, also, in another way. In the first part, values 'evident' in mental health legislation have been sought out, that is, the starting point of the analysis is the legislation. In comparison, in the latter parts of the paper, the starting point is more general value considerations and mental health legislation is used as an example of these values, particularly as an example of values relevant to medicine. Although, often, no matter which of these forms of analysis is undertaken the same range of values will be disclosed, this will not necessarily or always be the case. Further, it is worth mentioning that in undertaking both types of value assessment (and possibly this could be characteristic of a legal approach and, consequently, typical of lawyers), I have acted somewhat dogmatically in drawing inferences as to what value elements *were* responsible for *presently* observed facts. It is recognized that others may well caution more reticence in reaching some of these conclusions.

PART I. CHANGES IN MENTAL HEALTH LEGISLATION

The changes in fact

Changes have been made in both England and Ontario with respect to the grounds for involuntary hospitalization. In England, the requirement that certain groups of mentally disordered persons be treatable in order that they be detained, was added to the existing requirements that detention be necessary for treatment and in the interest of the health or safety of the patient or for the protection of others.[2] In addition, the durations of both initial detention and its subsequent renewal with respect to patients 'admitted for treatment' are halved by the Mental Health Amendment Act,[3] now the Mental Health Act 1983. Prior to the 1978 amending legislation in Ontario, requirements for involuntary hospitalization included a similar 'safety' standard to that presently in force under the Act in England.[4] Ontario has since adopted a more stringent 'dangerousness' standard, which essentially requires a likelihood of serious physical harm to the mentally disordered patient himself or to others.[5] Procedurally, the 1978 Ontario legislation adopts a process whereby a prospective patient is first held for a short-term 'assessment' period, during which it is determined whether involuntary hospitalization would be appropriate.[6] In contrast to the Ontario approach, the English Mental Health Act allows for the medical treatment of patients in the 'assessment' phase,[7] thereby establishing the nature of this period as being not only for diagnosis, but also for short-term treatment. It should be mentioned here that all periods of detention allowed under the Ontario Mental Health Act are much shorter than those specified in the English legislation.[8]

The English Act has had the effect of increasing patient access to Mental Health Review Tribunals which were established under the 1959 Act.[9] In addition, a system of automatic referral was introduced to ensure that all patients were provided with the safeguard of independent review.[10] In response to the 1981 decision of the European Court of Human Rights,[11] these tribunals were also given the power to discharge restricted patients (that is those held under criminal commitment procedures).[12] Similarly, the 1978 Ontario legislation introduced increased access to review,[13] a system of automatic review,[14] and, in addition, a right of appeal from a review board to a county or district court.[15]

In both England and Ontario, reform of the mental health legislation clarified the position of the psychiatric patient with respect to consent to treatment. In Ontario, informed consent to treatment by the patient (or nearest relative in the event of incompetency) is the rule.[16] However, the Act sets up a system for overriding refusal of consent which requires certificates by three professionals (the attending physician and two psychiatrists) and the intervention of the Ontario Review Board.[17] On the face of the legislation, it appears that England recognizes a system which allows for more extensive overriding of the patient's refusal of treatment. Certain treatment may be imposed where one medical practitioner[18] is of the opinion that it is necessary.[19] The English legislation also enacts emergency provisions which eliminate the need for consent in specified circumstances.[20] Finally the Act contains a provision which states that consent is unnecessary for any treatment not yet specifically mentioned in the legislation or regulations.[21]

Some new provisions in England reflect a concern that involuntary hospitalization only be resorted to when other possibilities, in the form of community and social services, have been exhausted. An Approved Social Worker, before making an application for involuntary hospitalization, must first satisfy himself that detention is the most appropriate way of dealing with the patient.[22] Then, subsequent to the admission of a patient admitted on the application of a *relative*, a designated social worker must interview the patient and furnish a report on his social circumstances.[23]

With respect to criminal offenders, the new English legislation introduced a system allowing remands of accused persons to hospital, thereby increasing the opportunity for psychiatric assessment and treatment of these persons.[24] Similar provisions exist, both provincially and federally, for dealing with such persons in Ontario.[25] The English Mental Health Act 1959 had established a 'hospital order' system for dealing with mentally disordered persons convicted of an offence.[26] The basic system remains essentially unchanged by the Mental Health Act 1983, but patients are given more extensive rights with respect to review of their detention and discharge.[27] Ontario is constitutionally barred from legislating such a system, because criminal law is a federal jurisdiction,[28] and the federal Criminal Code provisions do not deal adequately with the management of these persons.[29] It is not mandatory that such persons be hospitalized, rather than imprisoned, nor even that they be treated, and if treated the position with respect to consent to treatment is unclear.[30]

The changes in values and policies

What values and policies and what changes in values and policies do the legislative provisions governing 'civil commitment', outlined above, represent?

Grounds for involuntary hospitalization

Ontario law requires that, before a person can be involuntarily hospitalized, the attending physician must be of the opinion that the 'person is suffering from mental disorder of a nature or quality that likely will result in serious bodily harm to the person, . . . [or] to another person, or imminent and serious physical impairment of the person'.[30a] This can be interpreted as requiring in all cases, that the person be dangerous to himself or others, if 'dangerousness' is given a slightly extended meaning, as it is suggested it should be. Such an approach focuses all involuntary commitment decisions towards the same basic criterion of dangerousness, which, it is proposed, is desirable. The reason that there is some doubt with respect to the uniformity of the criterion underlying these alternative bases for involuntary hospitalization, concerns the last of them, which can be compared with the 'health or safety' bases for involuntary hospitalization of a person suffering from a mental disorder espoused in the English Act. The provision in the Ontario Act, however, is much more restrictive than that in the English statute and can be accommodated within a 'dangerousness' rationale. This is the case if it is regarded as applying to the situation in which the patient is dangerous to himself, but through 'lack of competence to care for himself'[30b] rather than from an overt act threatening bodily harm to himself.

There are also reasons against adopting this analysis. Involuntary hospitalization is an intervention by the state, through the agency of physicians, which interferes with the liberty of a person. Theoretically, such an intervention is justified under the state's 'police power' when it is based on dangerousness and under the '*parens patriae* power' (the power of the state, as a 'good parent', to protect those of its members unable to take care of themselves) when it is based on preservation of health. It may be important to identify the source of a power justifying a given intervention if the limits of the right to intervene are to be accurately determined. Thus, an intervention should not be justified under the police power if its true justification is the *parens patriae* power. In this respect, it can be argued that any interference with a decision of a person which concerns only himself should be based on the *parens patriae* power whether or not dangerousness is involved. Both the Ontario and English Acts include powers derived both from the police power and the *parens patriae* power. It is just that the initial focus on one or other of these two types of power and the overall balance between them may be different in the two jurisdictions. The Ontario Act appears to be more oriented towards the police power and the English Act towards the *parens patriae* power.

The approach taken in Ontario where there is at least a major, if not exclusive, emphasis on dangerousness, represents a general trend in formulating the basis for involuntary hospitalization in North America. At least on paper, such an approach appears more restrictive of involuntary hospitalization than the criterion formulated in the English Act, which, in looking to the health or safety of the patient or others, while including consideration of dangerousness, may in comparison with the Ontario Act be more welfare based.

Although it is stated above, it is worth pointing out expressly that in one important respect the English and Ontario legislation is the same: in both jurisdictions it is a condition precedent to involuntarily hospitalizing a patient that he be suffering from a mental disorder.[30c] The English and Ontario legislation is also similar in another important respect: in both jurisdictions the bases for involuntary hospitalization and the requirements surrounding the use of these provisions, indicate that involuntary hospitalization should only be used as a final resort.[31] Adoption of such an approach promotes a primary policy of treatment of mentally ill persons within the community or, when needed, by voluntary hospitalization.

One may question also, what the different bases for involuntary hospitalization reflect in terms of promoting a value of production of well-being – what is sometimes termed beneficence – as compared with one of avoidance of harm. In some situations where it may be justifiable to intervene to avoid harm, it may not be justifiable to intervene to confer a benefit.[32] Could it be that a 'dangerousness' criterion for involuntary hospitalization reflects principally a harm-avoidance value base and policy while a 'health and safety' one includes a wider spectrum of benefit-conferring elements?

The change to a more restrictive 'dangerousness' criterion for involuntary hospitalization reflects the greater hesitation that exists in relation to the use of this procedure today as compared with the past. There has been increasing sensitivity to the fact that involuntary hospitalization is the major exception in western societies to requiring criminal conviction in order to incarcerate a person. As such, it is a serious matter and that seriousness is no longer disguised or lessened, as may once have been the case, by the fact that it is a medicalized decision. Infringement of any person's liberty should only be possible in exceptional circumstances and where it is fully justified.

While the above is true, both the English and Ontario legislation leave a wide margin for professional judgment. For instance, whether conduct on the part of a mentally disordered patient is sufficient to fulfil the statutory definitions of 'dangerousness' can be debated, and whether 'dangerousness' can be predicted is the subject of much controversy.[33] In short, there is a need to distinguish between, on the one hand, the formulation of the law and the law in theory and, on the other, the interpretation and application of the law in practice. The two may be quite different. Such differences may also reflect that there are different values in theory and in practice, and different policies in theory and in practice.[34]

Some principles have been developed to explain these aberrations between theory and practice. For instance, Daube's principle of hidden mutilation proposes that we will accept mutilating a person if we are not constantly reminded that we have done so by being faced with the results.[35] Then there are theories, such as those concerning overt and latent decision-making,[36] which postulate that we will tolerate decisions which derogate from purportedly overriding values, for instance that of the sanctity of life, as long as those decisions and derogations are not overt.[37] Related to this theory are considerations concerning the allocation of risks: when risks appear to be imposed by chance a much higher level of risk, in terms of both probability and seriousness, is acceptable than when a risk is obviously imposed by choice.[38]

Relationship of criteria for entry to and exit from involuntary hospitalization

Not only the basis for imposition of involuntary hospitalization needs to be considered, but also the ease with which this can be instituted compared with the ease with which it can be reversed.

The possibilities with respect to ease of entry to and release from involuntary hospitalization are that: first, it is difficult for a person to be involuntarily hospitalized and difficult to be discharged; second, it is easy to be involuntarily hospitalized and easy to be discharged; third, it is easy to be involuntarily hospitalized and difficult to be discharged; fourth, it is difficult to be involuntarily hospitalized and easy to be discharged. The fourth of these options is the most protective of civil liberties in that it emphasizes values of respect for liberty, autonomy and self-determination. The third option is the least protective. It is suggested that possibly the Ontario Act most closely approximates the first option and the English Act the second. Each of these options constitutes a different compromise between the two extremes shown by the third and fourth options.

The rationale for suggesting that Ontario legislates a position of 'difficult entry' and England one of 'ease of entry' is outlined above in the discussion of the basis for involuntary hospitalization.[39] It is further suggested that Ontario legislation could, depending upon its interpretation, most closely represent a position of 'difficult discharge' and English legislation one of 'ease of discharge'. Leaving aside for a moment the rights to review of involuntary hospitalization legislated in both the English and Ontario Acts, one may compare other procedures for discharge provided under the two Acts. In England, the responsible medical officer, the hospital managers, and the nearest relative of the patient all have the power to discharge the patient.[40] The responsible medical officer and hospital managers may exercise their power of discharge at any time and no statutory criteria are applicable. The nearest relative has a similar power of discharge which can be 'barred' by the responsible medical officer only where 'the patient . . . would be likely to act in a manner dangerous to other persons or to himself'.[41] This is theoretically a stricter standard and more protective of the patient's liberty than that required as a basis for involuntary hospitalization. In contrast, the Ontario Act provides that '[a] patient shall be discharged [presumably by the attending physician] . . . when he is no longer in need of . . . observation, care and treatment'.[42] This is clearly a less stringent standard in terms of protection of liberty than that required in Ontario as a basis for involuntary hospitalization. However, it could be argued that 'dangerousness' is a continuing requirement if the involuntary hospitalization of a person is to remain justified, and that the provision for discharge must be interpreted in the light of this requirement. Alternatively, this discharge provision may be establishing that a duty to discharge an involuntarily hospitalized patient, as compared with his right to initiate proceedings to have himself discharged, only arises when he is no longer in need of care, rather than when he is no longer 'dangerous'.[43] However, quite apart from such difficulties of construction, all of the distinctions outlined above could be merely theoretical ones, depending upon the practical application of the various provisions, and taking into account the right to apply for review of involuntary hospitalization provided in both Acts.

Decision-making powers and procedures in mental health legislation[44]

Choice of decision-makers and procedures

A further factor is *who* decides, and according to *what procedures*, whether a person fulfils the criteria for involuntary hospitalization. The choice of persons and procedures again reflects certain values.

The English and Ontario mental health legislation has, on the whole, retained medicalization of the decision-making. This probably reflects a value of trust in the medical profession, a value that physicians are the most appropriate and best decision-makers in this context, and a view that fundamentally or predominantly it is a medical decision which is involved, or at least an area where the decision-making should be medicalized even if it has wider aspects.

There are, however, in both jurisdictions, aspects of decision-making concerning patients that have been either more judicialized (that is, courts or quasi-judicial tribunals or bodies are involved) or simply have been non-medicalized, in that persons other than physicians (but not courts) are required to be involved in the decision-making. What values or policies does this reflect? Does it show a distrust of the medical profession? It is suggested that this is not necessarily the case, and that unless there is good reason to believe that such an implication is true, it should be avoided. Rather, it constitutes recognition that there is a wider value base needed for some decision-making than that which can be provided only from the perspective of physicians. Unfortunately, however, many physicians do perceive such requirements as showing distrust of them. For instance, remarks made by physicians concerning some decisions of United States courts regarding non-prolongation of treatment of terminally ill persons exhibit such a belief.[45]

The procedures used for decision-making are necessarily related to the nature of the decision-maker. For example, different procedures can be required when a court is the decision-making body than would be possible in purely medical decision-making. However, some requirements, such as keeping a written record of the reasons for the decision, etc., can always be utilized.

There may also be mixed procedural–substantive requirements applicable to a given decision-making situation, such as the necessity of considering alternatives to involuntary hospitalization before this course of action can be justifiably adopted. Such requirements are often referred to generically as the rule mandating that 'the least restrictive and least invasive alternative reasonably available' be used. Hence, it is only when a more invasive and restrictive procedure is the only reasonable alternative that it may be employed. Detailed articulation of such standards can best be seen in relation to particular examples (for instance the standards that have been developed by courts and by bodies of enquiry such as Law Reform Commissions regarding the sterilization of mentally incompetent persons).[46]

Activating psychiatric assessment and involuntary hospitalization
Two important issues concerning the value placed on civil liberties are: first, how a person whom it is thought might need to be involuntarily hospitalized can be brought in for examination to determine whether or not he fulfils the necessary criteria; and, second, who can activate the issuing of an order for involuntary hospitalization.

In England an Approved Social Worker may in certain limited circumstances apply to a justice of the peace to obtain an order to convey a person to hospital for psychiatric examination.[47] The police also have the power to authorize detention for psychiatric examination of a person found in a public place who appears to them to suffer from mental disorder.[48] In Ontario, anyone may bring information on oath before a justice of the peace to seek an order for psychiatric assessment.[49] In addition, a police officer who feels it would be dangerous to proceed in the manner just described, has the power to take a person into custody for psychiatric assessment.[50]

Under the English Act, an application for short- or long-term involuntary hospitalization must be made by either the Approved Social Worker or the nearest relative, and must be founded on the written recommendation of two medical practitioners (one with psychiatric experience) who have examined the patient.[51] In Ontario, it is only a physician who has examined the person who can make an application for psychiatric assessment.[52] This application forms the basis for a second physician to examine and assess the person, following which that person may be involuntarily admitted to hospital.[53]

Again, there may be subtle differences in the values and policies reflected by the different ranges of persons who can instigate assessment or involuntary hospitalization procedures. For instance, excluding non-physician professionals and relatives from any formal role in initiating the process of involuntary hospitalization under the Ontario Act could be explained in several ways. The reasons could include a desire to make the decision appear entirely medical, or a desire to exclude either the possibility of vindictiveness or conflict of interest on the part of a family member, or, recriminations by the patient against that family member at some later date.

Decisions in emergency situations

One can compare also the emergency provisions in the English legislation with the non-inclusion of any such provisions in the Ontario Act. One such provision is that treatment can be administered without the need for the patient's consent or a second opinion in certain specified emergency situations.[54] Generally, the situations contemplated are those in which immediate action is necessary to prevent a life-threatening situation, serious deterioration, serious suffering, or violent behaviour.[55] Another emergency provision contemplates a relaxing of admission requirements in an emergency situation, such that the application need be founded on only one written recommendation of a medical practitioner who must, if practicable, have had previous acquaintance with the patient.[56] Emergency provisions may be able to be implied, but are not expressed, in the Ontario Act. Or could it be that the failure to include them in the legislation expressly, indicates a legislative intention to preclude their implication?

Rights to review of involuntary hospitalization

Under both the English and Ontario Acts, orders for involuntary hospitalization automatically expire unless renewed. Requirements for such renewal can be regarded as constituting one form of review of the continued detention of patients, and as review which must take place at certain specified times.[57] Patients are also given rights to apply for review.[58] To the extent that the rights to review of involuntary hospitalization in mental health legislation formulate a procedural due process requirement, it should be asked what values are demonstrated by such a requirement. Among these values are those of natural justice (the right to be heard and to have an impartial assessor) – fairness, reasonableness, openness, access to review, listening to both sides and access to a judicial or quasi-judicial tribunal.

It may be fruitful to examine this range of values in terms of whether it includes only individualistic values, or also integrative ones – what have been called the traditionally 'masculine', as compared with the traditionally 'feminine' values, respectively[59] – because it may not be sufficient to look at the mentally ill person simply as an individual; he may also need to be viewed within his social network of family, community and society. Difficulties arise when respecting individualistic values would be destructive of integrative values and vice versa. The law has not, in general, been as protective, if at all, of integrative values and, in fact, these have probably been less valued and regarded as of a lower moral order than individualistic values.[60] There is danger in promoting integrative values in that their predominance could cause the rights of individuals to be unjustifiably sacrificed. It is suggested that the key to avoiding this is to recognize that in situations of conflict between individualistic and integrative values, one must judge which will predominate from the point of view of what is best for the individual. It is quite different to promote, for example, the interests of a family because this is best for a given individual, than to do so because it is best for the other members of the family.

Another line of relevant enquiry is to ask whether there is a need for different considerations, principles and procedures when dealing with relationships between strangers as compared with relationships between intimates.[61] If there is, then a further issue is whether the medical relationship, in general, and the psychiatrist–patient relationship, in particular, should be treated as a relationship between intimates or a relationship between strangers.

When speaking of review, a further factor to consider is who carries out that review and whose interests a review tribunal represents. Does it represent the interests of the patient, or the community, or the medical profession, or all of these, in which case what does it do in situations of conflict? Mental health legislation needs careful analysis to determine what priorities it establishes in this respect. In particular, the composition of the review tribunal will be an important factor.

It is also worth noting the categories of person who can apply for review of an order for involuntary hospitalization or for discharge of the patient. During initial specified periods of assessment or treatment under the English Act, only the patient can apply for review,[62] whereas in Ontario the patient or any person acting on the patient's behalf may make such an application.[63] In England, the nearest relative has a right to discharge the involuntarily hospitalized patient, but this right is subject to being overridden by a 'barring certificate' from the responsible medical officer.[64] The nearest relative then has a right of appeal against any such certificate to the Mental Health Review Tribunal.[65] In Ontario, anyone can act on behalf of an involuntarily hospitalized patient to seek his discharge, but this right exists simply as part of the general right to seek review of a patient's involuntary hospitalization.[66]

What values or policies do these various degrees of restriction on third parties' rights to intervene on behalf of the patient represent? Does the restriction of rights to the patient in the English Act reflect a value of keeping out 'officious intermeddlers' in certain situations? Or does it, rather, reflect a medical value, a view that, unless the patient is well enough and motivated enough to apply for review, then probably his involuntary hospitalization should continue, especially as he can be discharged pursuant to either an application by his nearest relative, or the process of automatic review, which offers adequate protection against an indeterminate incarceration? Does restricting rights of application for review to the patient reflect medical reality, or does it fail to take into account the effect on the patient of the phenomenon of institution-alization?

This relatively small (although important) issue of who can apply for review demonstrates again that there is a need when formulating a policy to identify the values actually being promoted, and those it is sought to promote, and to balance harms and benefits of, and considerations and interests enhanced or inhibited by, alternative approaches.

Consent to or refusal of treatment
Confusion of involuntary hospitalization and consent
The issues involved in involuntary hospitalization have often been confused with those arising from the obligation to obtain the patient's informed consent to treatment and from the patient's right to refuse treatment. Sometimes, the source of the amalgamation of issues relating to involuntary hospitalization and consent to or refusal of treatment, has not been confusion, but a view that the only reason or justification for involuntarily hospitalizing a patient is in order to treat him; therefore, not only is it unacceptable to hospitalize compulsorily without treating, but also, compulsory treatment is authorized by the hospitalization. Almost universally, this approach has changed, and the two issues of involuntary hospitalization and rights regarding consent to or refusal of treatment, are now dealt with separately.

Overriding a patient's decision
The underlying values in requiring informed consent to and honouring a refusal of treatment are respect for the person and his rights of autonomy or self-determination and inviolability (that is, the right not to have one's physical or mental integrity interfered with without one's consent).[67] However, both the English and the Ontario mental health legislation provide for overriding a competent patient's refusal of treatment,[68] which

shows that autonomy is not regarded as being an absolute value.[69] The situations in which this may occur are more restrictive, and the conditions required are more stringent, in Ontario than in England. In particular, there is one crucial question of interpretation with respect to consent raised by the English Act. It could be argued that because the physician need not respect a patient's refusal of treatment during the first three months of treatment,[70] there is no obligation to obtain the patient's consent during this period. This would be the case if it were held that it is illogical to seek the consent of a person whose refusal need not be respected. However, it is submitted that such an interpretation should be strongly rejected and that the statute can be interpreted in accordance with such a rejection. The 'consent process' serves functions other than simply eliciting agreement: it involves a transfer of information to the patient. Access to such information is an important right of the patient, who should not be deprived of any more of his rights or to any greater extent, than is absolutely necessary. Further, because this provision in the Mental Health Act alters the common law, it should, according to usual rules of statutory construction, be interpreted in such a way that it does this to the least extent possible, in terms of depriving the patient of rights which he would otherwise have.

It is important to examine the ways in which a patient's refusal of consent to treatment may be overridden, because this demonstrates the relative value weight given to autonomy. It also demonstrates the relative value weight attributed to the competing value of beneficence, when autonomy conflicts with a perceived conferral of benefit on another person.[71] In this respect, it should be kept in mind that there is often no more dangerous situation in terms of breaching another person's rights, than when a claim is made to do so in the name of conferring benefit. One is more likely to be cautious oneself and to instill caution in others regarding one's conduct, when one is not purporting to confer benefit, than when one is.

Competence
The definition of competence and the distinction between competent and incompetent patients is difficult and complex in both theory and practice and is still being developed.

Partial and global competence. In the past, competence tended to be judged globally, and a person was held to be either competent or incompetent in all respects. This has changed. The more modern approach is to assess functional competence, that is to determine competence with respect to the particular function for which competence is required.[72] Such an approach contemplates both partial and global competence or incompetence. In the former case, a person can be competent to perform one function but not all functions.

Emotional and cognitive competence. There is a factor relevant to competence which has not, in general, been taken into account directly by the law in the past, and which is particularly important in the area of consent to or refusal of treatment in psychiatry: this is the issue of what could be called emotional competence.

The law has been more concerned with the presence or absence of cognitive competence. A difficult situation arises when a patient is cognitively competent (that is, the patient has 'the ability to understand the subject matter in respect of which consent is requested and is able to appreciate the consequences of giving or withholding consent')[73], but suffers from mental illness of a kind that causes him to have an emotional disorder which may affect his decision choice. Should the consent to or refusal of treatment by such a person be respected?[73a] As a practical matter, it is more likely that his refusal will be brought into question than his consent.

In this respect, it is worth noting that the more a patient's decision deviates from what the physician thinks he would have decided in the same circumstances, and the more serious the outcome of the patient's decision in terms of being a threat to his own life or health, the more likely it is that the patient will be judged incompetent.[74] It is necessary to recognize a competent patient's refusal of treatment and to be careful that such a refusal is not simply seen as an indication of, and basis for determining, a patient's incompetence, as has sometimes happened. What constitutes incompetence depends entirely on the term's definition. This can range from requiring that a patient simply be able to indicate a decision, to requiring a rational decision-making process or outcome or, even more stringently, that the patient has subjective understanding of the information on which the decision is based, before one can regard him as competent and his decision as legally effective.[75] It is a value and policy choice as to which definition is adopted and whether the same definition will be used in all circumstances.

Understanding and rationality. It is also suggested that the distinction between understanding and rationality on the patient's part is particularly important both in relation to assessing competence and as regards psychiatry in general. It should be enough if the patient *apparently understands* the information that he is given and acts upon.[76] A rational decision outcome is sometimes required as an element of competence in order that, in its absence, a patient's refusal of treatment can be overridden and another person's decision imposed. But there is little point in asking for the patient's decision if he cannot refuse. If consent is to have any meaning at all, the option of refusal must always be present and to deny recognition of a competent patient's refusal of treatment simply on the basis of irrationality, negates the primary purpose of requiring informed consent, that is, respect for the right of self-determination.[77]

Again, the choice of definition of competence would depend on the values a society wished to promote. If it were most concerned to promote autonomy, then it would choose the most lenient definition of competence. This would be simply that the patient is able to evidence a decision for or against any proposed treatment, no matter what information he understood or why he chose a particular option. On the other hand, if a society wants to promote beneficence above all else, it might use the most stringent definition of competence in order to override decisions which it feels would not promote the benefit of the patient and may, in fact, even do him harm. In between these two extremes a definition can be adopted which strikes some compromise between fully promoting either autonomy or beneficence.

Mechanisms for respecting autonomy of incompetent persons. Another matter which could be considered here is whether it is possible to devise mechanisms for respecting the autonomy of persons who have periods of incompetence. For example, if a person has lucid intervals it may be possible for him to make decisions during those intervals which would be applied when he becomes incompetent, or, at least, to choose his own decision-maker for those times.[78] This approach allows for a greater exercise of autonomy by the incompetent person and respect for his autonomy, than would an approach of imposing on him the decision of a stranger.[79] It is important to be aware of and sensitive to the need to develop such mechanisms. Perhaps this recognition is just commencing, in a formal manner, in the law, although, possibly, such procedures have been used on an *ad hoc* basis by medical professionals in the past.

Basis of decision-making for incompetent persons. A related matter is that of the basis of decision-making to be used with respect to incompetent persons. Again, there has been more precise definition in the recent past. Two possible bases are those of 'best interests' and substituted judgment.

'Best interests' is a more objective approach, where the third party decision-maker decides what is in the best interests of the incompetent person. Substituted judgment, on the other hand, can first of all involve a substitute decision-maker chosen by the incompetent person when competent, or, if no such choice has been made, a person who is likely to know what decision the incompetent person would have made were he able to decide. Members of the person's family are the most likely to fulfil this criterion, which is one reason for using them as substitute decision-makers.

There is, again, a difference in nuance in the values being promoted depending upon whether a 'best interests' approach or substituted judgment is adopted. There may also be policy implications, because a 'best interests' criterion allows wider scope for third party (including bureaucratic) decision-making than does substituted judgment. For instance, when substituted judgment is used, any statement that the incompetent person made while competent (for example, that he would not want to be given life-support treatment in certain circumstances), or any religious view (for example, concerning blood transfusions), and other subjective factors, would be more likely to be taken into account than they would be were a 'best interests' model of third party decision-making used. In short, a substituted judgment basis for decision-making promotes autonomy to a greater degree than does a 'best interests' basis.

Legislative definitions of competence. Other issues concerning competence can arise from its express or implied legislative definition. Competence is defined by implication in the English Mental Health Act[80] and is expressly defined in the Ontario Mental Health Act,[81] but this latter definition can be contrasted with that, for example, in the Ontario Mental Incompetency Act,[82] which is quite different. Does this simply reflect that competence is being assessed with respect to different functions that the patient must carry out, or for different purposes or circumstances, or could it be that when one compares the various statutes of a jurisdiction these contain inconsistent definitions?

Even when incompetence is defined, one must ask who is to judge competence and, in general, the statutes do not state this. But, almost certainly, it would be implied that it would be for the physician or the particular decision-makers authorized with respect to any decision or review, to judge. There is also the issue of whether there needs to be independent judgment or review of such findings of competence or, especially, of incompetence.[83]

Categories of treatment

The concept of categories of treatment is common to both the English and Ontario Acts. But the nature of treatments, and procedures for overriding a patient's refusal of treatment, in any given category, vary between the two jurisdictions. The Ontario Act is far more stringent in its requirements in all these respects. The English Act contemplates three categories of treatment: first, psychosurgery (and other treatment specified by regulations); second, electroconvulsive treatment and the administration of medicine (and other treatment specified by regulations); and, third, all other forms of treatment for mental disorder.[84] The Ontario Act legislates two categories of treatment: first, psychosurgery; and, second, other forms of treatment.[85] There is a complete bar on psychosurgery on involuntarily hospitalized patients in Ontario.[86] In contrast, in England, psychosurgery can be performed with the consent of the patient and a second opinion from three persons (one a doctor) as to the patient's competence and a second opinion from the physician as to the likely effectiveness of the treatment. These safeguards apply to voluntary and involuntary patients.

When one looks for reasons why a treatment is in the more or less restrictive category, it is apparent that the degree of invasiveness of the treatment, its seriousness, its irreversibility (in terms of its potential to change the patient and his behaviour and emotions on a permanent basis) and the degree to which it is experimental, are criteria indicating that it should not be given without, at a minimum, personal informed consent.[87] Psychosurgery is the prime example of such a treatment and probably warrants additional safeguards. On the other hand, it can be argued that to prohibit a treatment or to impose safeguards other than the informed consent of a competent patient is to restrict the patient's autonomy unjustifiably and to invade the privacy of physician–patient relationship. However, one's right to consent to interventions on oneself is not unlimited: it is governed by doctrines of public policy and 'public order and good morals' and pursuant to such doctrines some interventions are totally prohibited. Consequently, it would seem reasonable for the law to institute an intermediate class of treatments – those which are neither totally prohibited nor freely available just with informed consent, but which, because of their nature or dangers of abuse are subject to special safeguards.

The English Act also contemplates that medication can be given despite a competent patient's refusal of it during the first three months after initiation of medication, without even complying with the additional safeguard mechanisms specified by the Act for overriding a patient's refusal.[88] If the results of one investigation, that most refusals of treatment are within the first two weeks of hospitalization, are of general applicability, this provision could in practice eliminate most refusals of treatment.[89] There is also a need to know why patients who initially refuse treatment desist from this. Is it that they are acclimatized, coerced, manipulated, or adopt a different role after this time – for instance, conformity to either the institution, its staff, or even to other patients' requirements – so that their refusals become less likely? Or is it that after this time they 'see the light' and agree with the opinions of their psychiatrists as to what is best for them, namely the suggested treatment? A warning has been sounded with respect to the phenomenon of institutionalization in situations where 'therapeutic responsibilities [have] been diffused by the creation of a whole new generation of non-medically trained therapists . . ., [and] the social responsibility of the . . . physician has been attenuated by the development of a separate group of health professionals who are essentially administrators or are systems management personnel'.[90] 'The goal of therapy then, of treatment and of cure, is thus necessarily subordinate to that of smooth institutional function and of administrative priority. In view of the burgeoning mental-health bureaucracy, this may justly be termed the "politicization" of psychiatry'.[91]

Further, under the English Act certain treatments other than medication, designated by the Secretary of State may also be given despite a competent patient's refusal of them.[92] One of the most debatable treatments in this respect would be electroconvulsive therapy.[93] It would need to be asked to what degree this treatment had temporary or irreversible effects to decide whether it should be categorized in the same way as psychosurgery, on the one hand, or medication on the other. However, there may be only a difference in degree and not in kind between the seriousness, the irreversibility of effects and even invasiveness of medication as compared with, for instance, surgery. Some adverse drug reactions, such as tardive dyskinesia, can be just as irreversible, just as debilitating, just as serious and distressing, as the effects of surgery. In fact, a patient's perception of ill-effects may be even greater with regard to adverse reactions to psychopharmacotherapy than to those arising from psychosurgery. Does it make a difference that the irreversible effect is a necessary aim in psychosurgery and an unwanted or secondary effect in drug therapy? It should be asked what values one seeks to protect by imposing strict limitations on the use of psychosurgery. Is the primary aim to protect individual patients from psychosurgery or, rather, is it to protect members of society as a whole from the feeling of being threatened with the possibility of non-consensual interference with their mental processes in a rather dramatic and overt way? Is this another example of accepting latent, but not overt, derogations from a principle, in that interference with mental processes via drugs may seem to constitute a less direct and obvious derogation, than psychosurgery, from the principle of the inviolability of the physical and mental integrity of a person, which carries the right to be free from non-consensual interference?[94]

The English Act also contemplates that other forms of treatment[95] not specifically dealt with in the Act do not need consent. One would need to query what these are. For instance, it could be that behaviour modification falls within such other treatments. There is a continuum extending from, at one end, the experience of living – one general description of which could be behaviour modification – through, in the middle, usual forms of education, to, at the other end, deliberate, highly invasive, often unacceptable forms of behaviour modification techniques. It can be difficult both in theory and practice to draw the line between what are and are not acceptable techniques and, therefore, it is difficult to determine when the border-line is crossed. The law has developed concepts of coercion and undue influence to control what is unacceptable conduct in certain circumstances, for example in the contractual setting. However, these concepts would be of little use in regulating the use of behaviour modification techniques, because they operate only to annul legal relationships, which would be an irrelevant remedy. Further, even if the concepts of coercion and duress could be given more general applicability there may still be problems with their use. These concepts indicate a difference in degree, rather than in kind, between what is acceptable and unacceptable conduct, and it is frequently difficult to determine the limits in any given case, especially as they vary with all the circumstances.

There has been little legal development in protecting persons from non-physical intrusions such as behaviour modification techniques often represent. On the whole, criminal law protections, such as those prohibiting assault, require physical contact or harm before an offence is committed.[96] There has been some development in tort law of a remedy for negligently inflicted nervous shock[97] and there is the tort of intentional infliction of mental suffering.[98] But again these could well prove to be inadequate remedies, even assuming they were applicable, for wrongful use of behaviour modification techniques.

There is a need to take additional care to be sensitive to the presence of coercion or undue influence in the broader sense of these terms when one deals with especially vulnerable populations such as the mentally ill and the mentally handicapped. There have been some instances in Canada of the use of unacceptable behaviour modification techniques (aversive conditioning), particularly with mentally handicapped persons, which have been the subject of public concern and debate.[99] For instance, are restraint systems acceptable and if so, when and on what conditions? Is it acceptable to deprive mentally handicapped persons of food and allow them to suffer the pangs of hunger when they have thrown their food in a dining room? Is there something inherently objectionable about putting a rubber band on the arm of a mentally retarded person and snapping this band against the person's arm as a pain-punishment aversive stimulus? Is it more unacceptable to use an electric cattle prod? Are there some psychological associations – for example, the fact that a cattle prod is normally used to control animals, which could give rise to feelings that the use of these on mentally retarded persons is to treat them as animals – that make this unacceptable, rather than the inherent nature of the technique itself? These are all difficult questions which need, again, to be examined in terms of both overt and latent values, and symbolism, and precedent-setting effects, and risks and benefits, all of which factors are relevant in determining the conduct a society will allow and the conduct it will prohibit.

Misuse of powers under mental health legislation
Preventing abuse
Another matter which should be considered is the misuse of involuntary hospitalization procedures and what is needed to protect against their abuse. There is no absolute protection against abuse of powers, and legislation which creates powers cannot necessarily include adequate protections against abuse. In fact, it may not need to do so, because there may be adequate common law remedies available. It might also be that providing a statutory remedy for abuse of the powers given under a statute would limit, rather than expand, the range of potential remedies. This can occur where a statute does not expressly reserve the common law remedies and a court holds, as a matter of statutory interpretation, that the statute is meant to cover the field and to provide all available remedies and that, to this extent, it abrogates any common law remedies which would otherwise be available.[100] Such a result would, it is proposed, be most undesirable, especially in relation to remedies available for wrongful involuntary hospitalization.

Values protected by legal remedies
The primary common law remedy for any continuing, allegedly wrongful detention of a person is the writ of 'habeas corpus'. The writ is issued to

the custodian who must appear before the court on a very short return date, to show justification for the detention, failing which the court will order release of the person in custody. The priority given to the writ of 'habeas corpus' by the courts emphasizes the heavy value weight attributed to and protection afforded rights of liberty.

It is also worth looking at the values supported by the common law remedies of assault, battery, false imprisonment and negligence, which could be available for abuse of the power to involuntarily hospitalize a person.[101] The torts of assault and battery protect autonomy and inviolability, that is, the right not to be touched or to be threatened with being touched without one's freely given consent. The cause of action in false imprisonment provides a protection of liberty in the form of freedom of movement. This tort can be committed in one of two ways: by either physical false imprisonment or psychological false imprisonment. Psychological false imprisonment occurs when a person has reasonable grounds to believe, and does in fact believe, that his liberty would be curtailed if he tried to do other than what the person psychologically imprisoning him required that he do. This tort is a strong legal expression of the value accorded the liberty of the individual citizen and is one of the important protections of that liberty. However, like many legal remedies it acts retrospectively after a wrong is committed and not prospectively in order to protect the person from potential infringement of his liberty, except to the degree that the threat of litigation acts as an inhibition of one person infringing the liberty of another. The basic principle or value underlying liability to compensate in negligence is that a person should pay for damage caused through his fault, even though the damage was caused unintentionally, in the sense that there was no intention to harm.

The concept of medical malpractice

The psychiatrist must walk a fine line of professional judgment if he or she is to avoid legal liability in relation to involuntary hospitalization. Against this, it should be kept in mind that the law allows a range of acceptable decision-making through the concept of 'reasonable professional judgment', within which it grants immunity from legal liability to the psychiatrist. Medical malpractice occurs when a physician acts in a way that no reasonably competent physician in the same circumstances would have acted. Errors do not of themselves constitute medical malpractice. Legal liability is attached to those errors which a reasonably competent practitioner would not have made.

Legal liability can arise not only for wrongful involuntary hospitalization, but also for failure to involuntarily hospitalize a patient when a reasonable psychiatrist in the same circumstances would have done so. If the patient subsequently harms himself (for example, commits suicide) or another (for example, murders) the psychiatrist could be liable for damages. Moreover, legal liability can arise in the latter situation in another way: even if the psychiatrist is protected within the concept of reasonable professional judgment for not involuntarily hospitalizing a patient, he may have a duty to warn potential victims of the patient.[102] The imposition of such liability raises many complex issues, not least among them being problems of breach of confidentiality towards the patient in warning potential victims.

Just as wrongful failure to discharge a patient could give rise to legal liability for, for example, false imprisonment, so could negligent discharge. Discharge in circumstances in which no reasonable psychiatrist would have discharged the patient who subsequently harms himself or others, could be a basis for liability for private law damages or (as a very remote consideration) even criminal law liability, in some rare circumstances where the discharge showed wanton or reckless disregard for human life or safety.[103]

If, as is frequently alleged, there is a malpractice crisis in some jurisdictions, what values and policies does such a crisis reflect? Is it simply a desire to maintain professional standards, or has it some control or punitive aims? Or is it a risk distribution mechanism, in that a physician is much more likely to be insured than a patient and the patient can only be compensated if the physician is held legally liable? The alternative is to give compensation simply on the basis of damage, whether or not it was caused by fault on the physician's part – the so-called no-fault or strict liability system.[104] This may avoid the stigma of fault for the physician, although the imposition of liability on any basis may carry an implication of wrong-doing. Strict liability would also make compensation more readily available to the patient. On the other hand, it would probably increase the cost of compensation for physicians or the cost of insurance and hence the cost of medical care.

Mental health legislation and some prohibited grounds of discrimination
Age

It is interesting to note that the English 1959 Act was altered by the 1982 Amending Act to remove an age limit to the effect that 'minor disorder' patients could only be involuntarily hospitalized for long-term treatment if they were under twenty-one years of age.[105] Persons with such a disorder who are over this age may now be involuntarily hospitalized, provided a 'treatability' test – that is, that there is an expectation of benefit from treatment – is also fulfilled.[106] The change in this section may reflect increased sensitivity to the value of non-discrimination on the basis of age. The original section may also have reflected a view that it was more acceptable to be paternalistic with respect to young persons than adults.[107]

Mentally handicapped persons

The application of mental health legislation to mentally handicapped persons and the values and policies this reflects also warrants investigation. The definition of mental disorder in the English 1959 Act[108] remains unchanged in the Amendment Act and is broad enough to include a mentally handicapped person for limited involuntary hospitalization. The White Paper for the new Act makes it clear that it was intended that, in certain instances, the Act would be applicable to mentally handicapped persons.[109] However, it is unlikely that such persons would be detained under the long-term involuntary hospitalization provisions because, in order for this to occur, they would, among other requirements, need to be exhibiting 'impairment of intelligence and social functioning' associated with 'abnormally aggressive or seriously irresponsible conduct' ('mental impairment' or 'severe mental impairment').[110] In contrast, the Ontario legislation is much less likely to be applicable to mentally handicapped persons. Although they would fall within the definition of mental disorder, i.e. 'any disease or disability of the mind',[111] this would need to be associated with the likelihood of serious physical harm to themselves or others before they could be involuntarily hospitalized pursuant to the Act.

An issue which is related to involuntary hospitalization is the institutionalization of mentally handicapped children and also adults by their parents or caretakers. Clearly, such action is needed in some cases. But it has been increasingly queried, at least in Canada, whether institutionalization is justified in all of the cases in which it takes place. It may be that augmented consciousness of the need not to involuntarily hospitalize a person except according to rather stringent criteria, will affect the approaches and attitudes taken in general towards institutionalizing mentally handicapped persons.

Two recent Canadian cases may be of interest in the above respect. In one of these, Justin Clark, a young man who suffered from cerebral palsy and had been institutionalized by his parents when he was a young child, sought to leave the institution to join a group home in Ottawa.[112] His parents opposed his wishes. In order to prevent him from leaving the institution the parents applied for a court order for guardianship[113] which would enable them, as guardians, to make decisions regarding Justin's care and custody. The provincial court of Ontario refused the parents' request and held that Justin was free to make his own decisions, including one to leave the institution.

One issue which is raised by the Justin Clark case is the interface and overlap between legislation providing for involuntary hospitalization and general guardianship orders.[114] This issue is currently being tested in cases being taken under the Dependent Adults Act[115] (the guardianship legislation) and Mental Health Act (the involuntary hospitalization legislation) of Alberta.[116] One of the Alberta mental health facilities is arguing that involuntarily hospitalized incompetent patients in their facility can be treated without consent and therefore do not require guardians. The public guardian is arguing that the Mental Health Act imposes on the mental health facility a duty to offer treatment, but does not authorize it to treat without the consent of a duly appointed legal representative of an incompetent patient, particularly now that there is an Act, the Dependent Adults Act, which specifically outlines the due process to be followed when the law requires a legal, substitute decision-maker.[117] Clearly, incompetent patients would be afforded greater legal protection by having both Acts apply. The question is how feasible this is in practice and, at a technical legal level, whether there is found to be an implied legislative intention that this should or should not be the case. The English legislation avoids some of these problems. It establishes a mechanism whereby a second physician can certify the patient's incompetence and the likelihood of a given treatment being beneficial, in which case the treatment may be administered.[118] In contrast, the Ontario legislation allows the nearest relative to consent for an incompetent person.[119] The issue is not addressed of what would happen if the person had a legally appointed guardian and there were conflict between the guardian and the nearest relative as to whether or not to give consent. One could argue that, in accordance with the usual rules of statutory construction, the specific provision, that in the Mental Health Act giving the nearest relative the power to make this particular type of decision, would override the more general provision in the guardianship legislation. On the other hand, the appointment of a named guardian by a court could be regarded as the more specific provision and therefore take priority.

Another issue with respect to medical decision-making for incompetent patients is whether a guardian would be required for all such adult patients, whether or not they were involuntarily hospitalized, or only for chronically ill persons and not for acute-care patients who were not likely to remain incompetent.[120] It would be rather expensive, in terms of economic and judicial time costs, to require court intervention before treating any incompetent patient. It should be noted that guardianship law only applies to incompetent persons, and any overriding of a refusal of consent by, or treatment without consent of, a competent patient would have to be expressly or impliedly authorized by mental health legislation, or at least by a court.[120a] In this respect, and although it is obvious, it is worth noting that statutes authorizing compulsory treatment pursuant to involuntary hospitalization do not automatically apply to institutionalized, mentally handicapped persons.

A further issue relevant to institutionalized mentally handicapped persons has arisen in another Canadian case, where a health care worker in an institution for such people physically disciplined a mentally retarded adult by hitting him on the head with a spoon.[121] In defence to a charge of criminal assault, the mental health care worker pleaded that a mentally retarded adult is a child for the purposes of the Criminal Code provision which allows reasonable chastisement of children.[122] The Court of Appeal of Ontario overruled the trial judge in holding that the mentally retarded person was not a child and that the health care worker was not a teacher or person *in loco parentis* within the terms of the provision. The issue has just been ruled on by the Supreme Court of Canada, which upheld the Court of Appeal.[122a] This ruling necessarily delivers a message about how Canadian society views mentally handicapped persons. In particular, it shows that it is not prepared to condone, at least overtly, the common phenomenon of infantilization of handicapped persons. Although our laws regarding children are usually meant to give them additional protection as compared with adults, this is not always the case, as the provision of the Criminal Code just referred to demonstrates. Further, even protection does not confer only benefit, but also can cause harm: it is a matter of choosing between competing harms and benefits – which, again, is often a value judgment.

Scope of mental health legislation

The above discussion raises an issue which, on the whole, has not been adequately dealt with in relation to mental health legislation: that of the scope of any given piece of legislation. Moreover, as the Alberta cases referred to above demonstrate, the limits of one Act as compared with another are not always clearly delineated.

One recent example of doubt concerning the scope of operation of mental health legislation is that it has been questioned whether involuntary hospitalization provisions in the English Mental Health Act could be applied in a general medical context.[123] For example, could the Act be used to override a competent patient's refusal to continue with life-sustaining treatment? It has been argued that it was never intended that the Act should be applied in such a way. However, there is usually nothing in the terms of such legislation, apart from finding an implied legislative intention to this effect, and strict interpretation of conditions precedent to involuntary hospitalization, such as the presence of mental disorder, to prevent such an application.

Monitoring the application of mental health legislation

The review tribunals set up under both the English and Ontario legislation provide one level of monitoring of the application of that legislation. But the English Act is notable in that it sets up an independent, large (ninety-member), transdisciplinary, monitoring and advisory body, namely the Mental Health Act Commission.[124] The Commission is empowered to visit hospitals, keep under review any aspect of care and treatment – which appears to be a wide mandate – and advise regarding patients' complaints and civil rights and the mental health care system in general. In particular, and possibly most importantly in terms of the general effect it will have, the Commission is to submit proposals for the 'Code of Practice' required to be drawn up under the Act.[125]

As far as value and policy analysis is concerned, the Commission represents, among other things, a recognition of the need for the input of community values into, and community involvement in supervision of powers given under, mental health legislation. Further, there is recognition that if the Commission is going to fulfil, and be seen as effectively fulfilling, its monitoring tasks, it must be independent and transdisciplinary and composed of a membership which will cause it to win respect for its opinions from a broad spectrum of the community and professions. The principal danger in establishing such an institution is that it constitutes a reassurance that all necessary protective measures are being taken and, to the extent that this is not true, patients could well be less protected than if no safeguard mechanism had been established. It is suggested that it would be most fruitful to undertake research in relation to the role and effectiveness of the Commission, particularly regarding the group dynamics displayed in both its internal and external operations and how decision outcomes are established.

'Criminal commitment' and values

The English Mental Health Act deals with both involuntary civil and criminal commitment,[126] that is, involuntary hospitalization pursuant to both civil and criminal processes. In comparison, in Ontario, criminal commitment is dealt with mainly under the federal Criminal Code,[127] whereas involuntary civil commitment falls under provincial law. Apart from the fact that historical accident can be regarded as the cause of criminal law being a federal jurisdiction and health law a provincial one, does this difference in dealing with these two types of commitment in Ontario as compared with England reflect or, perhaps more importantly, give rise to, different value and policy approaches as between the two forms of commitment? Could it be that treating both civil and criminal commitment in the same statute results in greater identification of mentally ill persons committed criminally with mentally ill persons committed civilly and, as a result, treatment of criminally committed persons primarily as mentally ill persons and secondarily as criminals, rather than vice versa? The order of identification adopted could affect decision outcomes because the primary identification is likely to be treated as determining the governing rule and the secondary identification as establishing the exception.[128]

The issue of 'criminal commitment' is a complex one. The value balance is different from civil commitment, because protection of the public is a much more dominant consideration. This is especially true when one is dealing with a mentally ill person who has been convicted of a criminal offence. The latter is not always the case, because a person can be diverted into the mental health care system prior to conviction, either because he is unfit to stand trial (when he is held under criminal commitment) or because a psychiatrist civilly commits a person who has been charged with an offence but not faced trial, and, in so doing, diverts him out of the criminal process.[129] When such a person is held under a civil commitment order the same rules apply as for any other civil commitment. However, when a person is held under criminal commitment, that is a hospital order, different rules apply both in England and in Ontario. These rules allow hospitalization for an indeterminate time by means of a 'restriction order' under the English legislation[130] or a Lieutenant Governor's Warrant under the Canadian Criminal Code.[131] The classic example of a person who will be criminally committed is the offender who pleads a successful defence of insanity.

On the whole there is not the same degree of concern attached to, and often there is felt to be more justification in, incarcerating and prolonging the incarceration of a person who has been charged with or, even more so, convicted of a criminal offence, as compared with one who has not. This difference in attitude towards persons held under criminal commitment is not only reflected in mental health legislation,[132] but also has other ramifications in that there may be less concern for the rights of criminally committed persons than those who have been civilly committed. Although this attitude is undesirable, it is necessary to keep in mind that judges and juries need to feel convinced that persons they subject to criminal commitment will not too readily be set at liberty. In default of such reassurance there may be reluctance to use criminal commitment procedures, with the result that mentally ill accused or convicted persons will probably be worse off. Nevertheless, the provisions applying in the criminal sphere which allow prolonged hospitalization on the basis of mental illness or incapacity have been the subject of abuse. In one Canadian case, a young man was incarcerated at the age of eighteen for an alleged offence of purse-snatching for which he was charged but not convicted. He was held on the grounds that he was unfit to stand trial. He was discovered by the Canadian Association for the Mentally Retarded seventeen years later, during which time he had been a continuous inmate of a maximum security institution for the criminally insane.[133]

The 'mental illness' provisions in the Criminal Code are currently under review in Canada and one aim is to draft laws and regulations which will at least inhibit, even if it is not possible totally to prevent, abuses.[134] In this respect, the major considerations should be to ensure that criminals who should be dealt with by the penal system rather than treated in the mental health care system are excluded from the latter;[135] to establish an adequate system for automatic review of the detention of criminally committed patients; and to give them proper opportunity to instigate review of their detention. All of these aims have been taken into consideration in the English legislation. One further factor which should also be dealt with is to ensure that criminals who ought to be taken out of the penal system and treated in the mental health care system have adequate access to the latter.

It may be of interest to note that the United States Supreme Court was recently called upon to consider whether 'hospital orders' for criminally convicted persons could exceed the maximum period for which those persons could have been imprisoned for the conviction.[136] The court held that the basis of incarceration when mental illness was present was dangerousness and that, therefore, the criterion for release was that the person was no longer dangerous. The argument was rejected that a person should be released when he had served time in a hospital equivalent to the maximum time for which he could have been incarcerated in a prison.

The very difficult issue of medical treatment of prisoners and their consent to treatment also arises in this context. It is suggested that the basic value and policy must always be to respect prisoners as persons and to honour their rights as far as possible. This means that rights which would not be contravened in a non-prison population can only be overriden where this is necessary because of the context of imprisonment. Consequently, prisoners should have the same rights to refuse treatment as other persons except when their refusal threatens the well-being of other prisoners, as for instance it would in relation to infectious disease.[137] The situation with respect to consent to health care by prisoners is, in general, a difficult and controversial one. It becomes additionally problematic when a prisoner is also mentally ill or criminally committed. In England, as far as consent to treatment is concerned, prisoners who are governed by the Mental Health Acts come under the same provisions as non-prisoners. This is not true for Ontario, where there is a great deal of doubt regarding this matter.

The concept of attributing the same rights to prisoners as are enjoyed by other members of our society, but regarding the exercise of some of these rights as being curtailed by the reality of imprisonment, may be helpful in achieving an approach and attitude towards prisoners which, it is suggested, is desirable. It may be thought that no matter what nice theoretical distinctions are made between various approaches, it makes little difference in practice which theory is adopted. While this is often true, there is a danger of depersonalization of prisoners if they are viewed as being rightless, and the approach suggested may help to overcome this.

There may also be situations in which the considerations and the relative values are not the same for prisoners as they would be for others. For instance, when a prisoner refuses treatment in order to manipulate the prison system the refusal of treatment may not carry the same weight that it would if the person were not a prisoner and were not refusing for such a reason. An American prisoner recently refused haemodialysis (without which he would die within a short time from the terminal renal failure from which he suffered) in order to seek transfer to another prison institution. The court held that he had not refused the treatment; he had agreed to dialysis but had simply refused the setting in which it was to be given, and that it was not open to him to refuse this.[138]

A related issue is hunger strikes in prisons. Again, the state's interest in force-feeding prisoners may be different from what it would be in relation to non-prisoner hunger-strikers. Are the applicable values or their weights different in relation to persons who have been placed deliberately in situations where their options are limited? Does it make a difference that refusal of either medical treatment or food is being used as a manipulative technique and that other techniques are not available because of the situation in which these persons have been placed?[139] Is it 'cruel and unusual treatment' to force-feed a prisoner, as was argued in one recent Canadian case?[140] How does force-feeding prisoners correlate with values being expressed in right-to-die movements and the controversy raging around withdrawal of life-support treatment, especially of artificial feeding?[141] These are general medical treatment issues, but the precedents they set could have profound effects in relation to treatment of prisoners and their mental health care.

In short, as this brief consideration of the values and issues related to prisoners' health care and treatment illustrates, changes in the circumstances in which values must be evaluated and placed in order of importance – for instance a prison as compared with a non-prison setting – alter the decision outcome.[142]

PART II. GENERAL CONSIDERATIONS UNDERLYING VALUES AND POLICIES IN MENTAL HEALTH LEGISLATION

In the first part of this paper the investigation started from an identification of the factual reality which exists and the changes which have taken place under mental health legislation. The values and policies represented by this factual reality and these changes were then speculated upon. In this second part, the investigation starts from the other end-point, that is, a consideration of some features of values and policy, both as general concepts and in some identified areas relevant to mental health legislation. The aim is to articulate the insights that these considerations can provide in relation to the values and policies underlying mental health legislation and changes in it.

The nature of values
Definition of politics, policies and values

The shortest definition of *politics* is that it is the art of the possible. *Policy* is defined in the *Oxford English Dictionary* as 'a course of action adopted and pursued by a Government, party, ruler, statesman, etc.; any course of action adopted as advantageous or expedient (the chief living sense)'. *Value*, again defined by the *Oxford English Dictionary*, in the sense of ethics, is 'that which is worthy of esteem for its own sake; that which has extrinsic worth'.

In one sense, it can be stated that it is impossible not to have a policy, not to have values, because a policy of not making decisions is itself a policy and exhibits certain values. In short, one cannot avoid policy and values: it is a matter of identifying, articulating, assessing, and, in cases of conflict, choosing between or reconciling them. Moreover, there is a need to assess whether one's policies implement one's chosen values. There may be unidentified inconsistency. This can occur when overt and latent values do not really coincide.[143] One obvious example of this is where a society proclaims an overriding value of the sanctity of life, as most societies do, and yet, in practice that society chooses not to do everything possible to protect and prolong life. For example, in England haemodialysis has not been routinely provided for all patients with terminal renal failure, in some hospitals when the patient is aged over sixty years and in others over sixty-five years.[144] Similarly, the treatment of defective newborn babies in both England and Canada almost certainly does not fully uphold a sanctity of life principle. Such hidden conflicts can cause, for instance, what a health care professional regards as a proper decision in a particular case to be strongly disapproved of by members of the general public. What may have occurred in such situations is that the health care professional has applied the latent principle and the general public the overt one.

Values in theory and in practice

The issue of latent values raises the question of how to reconcile what is ideal in theory and what is possible in practice.

Care needs to be taken that law, or rules, or guidelines, or recommendations are not brought into disrepute by having them ignored or, even worse, openly contravened, which is more likely when they are very difficult to fulfil. It has been suggested previously that, on face value, the Ontario Mental Health Act appears to be inclined towards more extensive respect for patients' rights than the English Act.[145] But does the English Act better reflect medical realities in practice than the Ontario Act? Law cannot be based just on theoretical notions, even when these notions are as important as those of fundamental human rights; it must also be workable in the arena of everyday life. It can be a fine line between using law to change attitudes and values, and enacting laws which are so far removed from present attitudes and values and practice that they are ignored and the law is brought into disrepute. This can be harmful in terms of the law's overall function of protection of persons, because it may cause other laws to be ignored when this would not otherwise have occurred.

Real as compared with theoretical change

Another question is whether changes in mental health legislation really represent changes in values or policies, or whether they may only appear to do this – what has been called 'innovation without change'.[146] This question needs to be examined both at a theoretical and a practical level, and it could well be that the answer will be different at each level. In other words, although in theory there may be the appearance of change of values, when the way in which the law is implemented in practice is examined, it may be apparent that this is not the case.

However, even if change in values only occurs at a theoretical level, it may increase sensitivity to the necessity of identifying underlying values and may increase self-criticism, which can lead to real change. It can be that the process of analysing an issue is as important as the practical decision outcome reached with respect to that issue. That is, although two identical courses of conduct may be undertaken in certain circumstances, the decision to act in this way may have been arrived at as a result of a different decision analysis. Recognition of this difference is important in terms of precedent-setting effect, because in future decision-making, depending on which analysis is used, the decision outcome may not be identical.

Further, this augmented sensitivity and self-criticism and awareness with respect to how decisions are arrived at, is becoming increasingly important, as there is increasing disagreement about moral aims in medicine and increasing pluralism in our societies in general. More precise analysis will be needed in order to choose and justify a decision choice when more people disagree with that choice.

Values concealing hidden conflicts

It may also be that value arguments are used as a cover for hidden conflicts. For example, inter-professional power struggles may be taking place in some confrontations centring on value conflicts. For instance, patients' rights can be used as a mechanism by non-physician health care professionals for challenging the power, exclusivity of practice and monopoly of physicians.

Linking of values

It may be that some values are seen as necessarily linked with others. There could be danger in this, in that if one of a pair of values is abrogated, so might the other be, when this is not a desirable outcome. For instance, the value of caring may be seen as being necessarily linked to paternalism and, therefore, the danger in lessening paternalism is to detract from the value of caring. Are autonomy and responsibility for oneself linked? If so, is there a tendency, in a more autonomy-based system, to say that it is the patient's fault that he is sick, especially where the illness is viewed as self-inflicted or the patient refuses treatment? Not least among the problems this could create would be that of guilt on the part of the patient, if he is told that he is responsible for his own illness. The creation of such guilt could be anti-therapeutic and a cause of additional suffering in some circumstances. Consequently, care would need to be taken that any risk of engendering guilt is justified.

Are values relative or absolute?

It is also relevant to consider whether there are any absolute values or whether all values must be judged in relation to the situation and circumstances in which they are applicable – the so-called situational ethics approach.[147] Is it correct to think that it is possible to have at least an absolute rule of *primum non nocere*, that is first do no harm, or is even this rule relative if it is accepted that it may be necessary to do harm in order to confer benefit and that acceptable conduct is to be judged simply as a matter of risk–benefit analysis and balance? These are complex philosophical issues which cannot be explored here, but it is necessary to be aware of them. The issue is whether there are any absolute rules which will function as satisfactory guides, provided that one restricts oneself to situations where one has only intentions of conferring overall benefit.

Values in relation to some specified areas relevant to mental health legislation
Values and language
Meaning

It is often a value judgment what content of meaning will be given to a particular term. For example, different language is chosen to define the criteria for involuntary hospitalization in the English and the Ontario mental health legislation, but it is necessary to inquire whether, in practice, the terms used are interpreted as applying to different situations so that, for instance, somebody could be involuntarily hospitalized under the English Act who could not be under the Ontario Act.[148]

Further, as noted, both the English and Ontario Acts provide for assessment of a potential patient, but under the English legislation this really amounts to a form of short-term involuntary hospitalization for treatment, whereas under the Ontario legislation it is simply a matter of psychiatric examination. Thus, the same word may envisage very different concepts and care must be taken in comparative studies to avoid confusion arising from the use of similar language which is given dissimilar meaning.

Complexity

There is also a question to be asked about the complexity of the language that is chosen. On the whole, the language used in the English Act is more complex than that in the Ontario Act and one may well ask why. It could be that this is a cultural reflection, or simply different drafting techniques. On the other hand, there may be more subtle reasons. For instance, the exemption in the English Act from needing consent to treatment during the first three months of treatment is drafted in a particularly complicated way.[149] One explanation for adopting such a style would be that the legislation is intended to establish an initial presumption that a patient's consent to treatment is required and then to allow an exception to this fundamental initial presumption, in that, in some circumstances, consent is not needed. If this were the reason that a complex drafting style was adopted, then it was chosen in order to promote the right to autonomy and self-determination. On the other hand, an alternative explanation is that complex language and style are being used in order to conceal, to some extent, the fact that consent is not needed in certain circumstances. Depending on which of these motives is the real one, very different underlying values and policies are being espoused. Similarly, one can query the motive for the use, in the English Act, of the term 'assessment' to describe the period during which the patient will not only be evaluated but also can be subject to short-term treatment.

Labelling

Language is not neutral.[150] The language that one chooses to use can be facilitative of certain courses of action, reflects values and attitudes and can have a 'labelling effect',[151] in that it can create attitudes and alter conduct towards persons who fall within its terms. In particular, there is often stigma attached to having been designated as mentally ill and, even more so, involuntarily hospitalized.

Further, it may be that once a label is attached, for instance a decision is made to involuntarily hospitalize a patient, it has a certain psychological and continuing effect on subsequent decisions. What is being suggested is that in a neutral situation, that is where there has been no label attached to a patient, an independent observer may classify or treat a patient differently from the way he would had the patient already been labelled.

Within this same context, other language and labelling factors affecting decision-making should be considered. For example, describing a decision option as being one of an 80% chance of benefit, rather than a 20% risk of failure, can affect a decision-maker's choice.

Communication

A prime purpose of language is communication, although it can, on occasion, also be used with a contrary aim when it operates as an exclusory device. More extensive 'communication rights' of patients than existed under prior legislation have been recognized in both the English and Ontario mental health legislation, reflecting a trend in medicine in general. However, the particular rights promoted are not the same in each jurisdiction.

These rights include the development of the doctrine of informed consent, which has probably caused physicians to inform patients more fully concerning the consequences and risks of treatment. A related issue is that of a patient's right of access to his medical records. The English Act, in contrast to the Ontario legislation,[152] does not provide for this. On the other hand, in England, unlike Ontario, there is a requirement that the patient and, except where the patient requests otherwise, his nearest relative be informed of the rights of the patient which exist under the English Act.[153] Further, this Act also provides that the nearest relative be advised of the patient's pending discharge, at least seven days in advance.[154] Finally, in both England and Ontario, most limitations on correspondence to and from patients have been removed.[155] This constitutes not only a recognition of the 'communication rights' of individual patients, but also provides an important safeguard in the implementation of all rights of patients and their overall protection. It is too easy to have 'paper recognition' of rights which are without practical effect. It is always necessary to think beyond simply recognition to implementation and how this can best be achieved.

Values and economics

A further question is whether some of the current trends to limit involuntary hospitalization are motivated by a desire to respect the liberty, autonomy and self-determination of patients, or to reduce costs and reallocate scarce resources. These latter considerations are proper and desirable aims; the question is when they should be predominant values. Further, it may be that treatment of mentally ill persons in the community is more expensive than in hospitals.[156] If this proves to be true, will there be a swing back towards easier and more frequent imposition of involuntary hospitalization? The answer is more likely to be affirmative if a major part of the impetus for dehospitalization is economic.

Values and medicine
Mental illness as a value judgment
The question of what constitutes mental illness has been asked with increasing frequency and vociferousness. There are certainly value elements involved in determining this, including in the scientific, medical and socio-political judgments involved.[157] One reason why this question has become more prominent is almost certainly the gross abuses of psychiatry in some countries in which 'therapy' has become applied politics. However, even when there is agreement as to what constitutes mental illness, there may not be as to what should be done about it, and a broader value base than just that of physicians may be needed in determining this. In this respect, it has been suggested that the provisions in the English Act, which require a social worker to assess that detention is the most appropriate way of providing the care and treatment a patient

needs,[158] 'show a recognition that compulsory admission to hospital involves not only a medical examination but also a social assessment'[159] of the patient.

It is also interesting to note that the English Mental Health Act, unlike the Ontario legislation, classifies mental illness into minor and major disorders[160] and, depending on which is diagnosed, different degrees of interference with the patient's liberty or inviolability are authorized.[161] This represents a policy of classifying the patient not only according to his conduct and his needs in terms of treatment but also according to his illness. Additional classification can be used to achieve more precise analysis of a situation and hence ensure that any action taken is justified. On the other hand, one needs to be careful that more interventionist approaches are not authorized simply on the basis of labelling, and that this is not used to conceal the absence of other necessary justifications.

Values and rights to health care

Another, contrasting issue which is raised, especially in the context of a discussion of involuntary hospitalization, is the right *to* health care. This can be distinguished from rights *in* health care, which have been the subject of much of the discussion throughout this text. Further, the above discussion has been concerned with the limits to be placed on imposing mental health care treatment without a patient's consent or where a patient refuses it. The contrasting issue which needs to be considered is whether there are obligations to provide health care when a patient requests it. In countries such as Canada and England, which have socialized health care systems, there are limits to the amount of resources that can be allocated by a government to medical care, and scarcity of medical resources has become an increasingly obvious and difficult problem. However, these socialized systems, in comparison with the private health care systems which predominate in the United States, do establish certain rights to health care, although these are not unlimited.[162]

The issue of rights to health care does not only depend on allocation, although it is most readily and frequently noticed in this context; it is also determined by geographical and psychological accessibility. Further, access to health care can also be an issue after a treatment relationship has been established, and physicians are usually the main factor in determining any given patient's access.[163] It has already been questioned whether the principal motivation behind dehospitalization of mentally ill persons is to reduce costs or respect rights.[164] Whatever the motivation, one effect of a general policy of dehospitalization could be to limit access to mental health care.

In terms of the current discussion, the relevant issue is the difference in underlying values that differences in allocation of and accessibility to health care reflect. They may well reflect some of the most important and fundamental values of a society, because attitudes towards provision of health care, particularly for the most needy and least powerful members of any society, have far-reaching ramifications.

Values and legal liability for failure to provide medical care

The above discussion also raises the issue of whether there are different principles applying to, and values activated by, acting or entering a relationship as compared with a situation of pure omission – whether to act or to enter into a relationship with legal implications. The common law has traditionally adopted an approach that, unless there is a pre-existing duty relationship, a person owes no duty until that person intervenes in a situation; that is, there is no legal liability, although there may be moral blame-worthiness, for a 'mere' omission. Civil law, by comparison, is more inclined to impose liability for pure omissions. For example, the French Penal Code[165] has been used to impose liability on physicians for omissions to give treatment in situations where the physician was not in a pre-existing treatment relationship with the patient.[166] It would only be if such a relationship already existed that a physician could be liable at common law for a wrongful omission to treat.

There are ancient legal precedents supporting the approach of the common law. Consequently, it may be argued that this approach is adopted simply as a result of historical accident and that it has not been changed because it is consistent with current societal values. But could it be that there are psychological reasons explaining this distinction in the common law between acts and omissions? For instance, could it be that one has stronger psychological bonding to a person with respect to whom one has intervened in some way, than to a person to whom one has done nothing; and does this result in a feeling of greater personal responsibility in the former situation which finds legal expression in the law's distinction between liability for acts and for omissions?[167] To what degree do such factors need to be taken into account in determining how involuntarily hospitalized persons should be treated? Does the fact that a physician has hospitalized a person make him more inclined to continue to treat the patient in some way, even if only by continued hospitalization?

Hospitalization as treatment

In this respect, it is proposed that hospitalization itself forms part of treatment and, consequently, any major change in a patient's hospitalization should be with the patient's informed consent. This proposition can be a source of difficulty and there are exceptions to requiring a patient's informed consent to change in his hospitalization, such as statutory rights to discharge patients who no longer need hospital care or special provisions applying to criminally convicted persons. But it is an important concept, because institutionalized persons can sometimes be dealt with primarily in terms of the physical space which they are permitted to occupy, more as though they were commodities than persons. Looking upon hospitalization as an element of treatment may help to overcome the development of such an attitude.

Values and policies of social control

Involuntary hospitalization raises the issues of social control and social conformity. Controls can range from being informal and non-institutional to formal and institutional; it is worth noting that the former can also constitute a form of control, although less obviously than the latter.

Social control can be viewed either as a means of bringing about a more desirable state of affairs in a society or as an end in itself.[168] In the former case, its purpose may be seen as holding together a social structure, when it will tend to be assessed in terms of its effectiveness in achieving this end – that is, in terms of its functioning.[169] When social control is seen as an end in itself, it is the process involved in control which will need to be justified, rather than its ultimate purpose. It has been proposed that in the latter case social control will be seen as involving the distribution of power, as motivated by self-interest, that formal rather than informal mechanisms will be emphasized, and that control strategies will not necessarily be either benevolent, or reforming, or part of a societal consensus.[170]

Involuntary hospitalization is an example of the latter type of social control. Thus, 'when an individual is defined as mentally ill and committed to an institution, it is the actions themselves, and their consequences, that must be accounted for'.[171] In contrast, approaches such as community mental health programmes fall within the former category of social control and would be assessed in terms of how well they function to bring about a desirable state of affairs. However, as there would need to be a consensus on what would constitute a desirable state of affairs, '[i]t has been suggested that such a view of social control is unrealistic, and it requires programs like CMH [Community Mental Health] to be evaluated by their performance in attaining an unreachable goal'.[172]

Analysis such as that outlined above may well be important in identifying the values and policies related to power and control that are being promoted by using certain approaches as compared with others in relation to mental health care. Perhaps even more importantly, it could assist in identifying the values and policies related to power and control which should be *avoided* in that arena.

Disvaluation

The final general issue to be addressed is that of disvaluation: adverse events may be more disvalued (that is, greater negative weight given to them) when they have not been experienced than when they have. For instance, a person may disvalue blindness more before he becomes blind than after this occurs. This is a relevant factor when considering the matter of third party decision-makers for incompetent persons. Most importantly, in the present context, the fact of incompetence may have a greater disvalue for someone who is not incompetent than someone who is. In short, one values situations differently depending on one's status *vis à vis* those situations.

Further, there may be some universal disvaluation factors. For example, it may be that risk is differently weighted or valued by aged persons as compared with younger ones. When older people were given a choice of decision outcome, one of which included a no-risk option, they usually chose this option, whereas younger people often chose risk-taking options which also promised greater benefit. On the other hand, when all available options involved risk, older people were no more likely than younger persons to choose the least risky one.[173] That is, a person's apparent values, as demonstrated by this choice among alternative options, may be altered by the decision-making framework which he is offered.[174]

PART III. THE STRUCTURE IN WHICH MENTAL HEALTH CARE POLICIES OPERATE

In this third section, some of the pillars of the underlying structure within which mental health legislation operates and within which it is implemented as policy, are examined. The areas chosen are: the relationship of medicine and law; the nature of professions; and principles relating to decision-making.

The role of law in relation to medicine

Relationship of medicine and law

An eminent Australian judge once said that 'law [is] marching with medicine, but [law is] in the rear and limping a little'.[175] It is not improbable that many physicians have wished that it would limp quite a lot more, if not become totally incapacitated. The law, among its other purposes, is an instrument for reflecting, upholding, creating and changing a society's values. These functions may occur at different levels. In this respect, law can be compared with the unconscious, conscious and super-ego of individual persons. Thus, the law may have unarticulated, unidentified and unexpressed purposes, sometimes, perhaps, even unknown ones; the 'black letter law' can be regarded as the law's conscious function (often the only one that most people recognize); and then one can look to the law's symbolic effect, which can be particularly important when one is trying to identify the values that the law is promoting or inhibiting. All these levels of functioning of the law are relevant to its relationship with medicine.

A historical aspect of the relationship of medicine and law

There is a universal trend for the law to be more involved in health care and in mental health care. This trend is not unique to any jurisdiction and is not necessarily indicative of problems in either just one society, or one profession, or one section of the medical profession, such as psychiatry. Further, with respect to any negative feelings generated by law's involvement in psychiatry, there may be some consolation, and perhaps interest, in noting that psychiatry was first taught as a part of what used to be called 'medical jurisprudence' in the medical curricula of the late nineteenth and early twentieth centuries. Thus, in one respect the teaching of law opened up the teaching of psychiatry in medical schools and this historical symbiosis could be a precedent for fruitful, creative, constructive and, one would hope, at least non-destructive interaction, in the future. Further, this cross-pollination has not only taken place in one direction. The teaching of aspects of psychiatry is opening up the teaching of law. This is particularly true in relation to modern criminal law.

Increased involvement of law in medicine

One question which arises here is why the involvement of law in medicine has increased. In the North American context, one could refer to the general increase in litigation in our societies, and to bureaucratization of, and regulation and government involvement in, a wide range of activities, all of which tend towards the increasing use of law. The involvement of law in medicine could be regarded as simply one example of this general trend. There is no doubt truth in this view. But there are almost certainly other relevant factors, including changes in the nature of professions and professional relationships.[176]

The protective and humanitarian functions of law, particularly with regard to highly vulnerable persons, are also relevant here. It is increasingly recognized that the sick, especially those who are mentally ill or dying or old, may have increased vulnerability. In the past, the personal professional relationship between the physician or health care professional and the patient and his family, and even between an institution, such as a hospital, and those it sheltered, was protective in a way that our modern professional relationships are not. Modern professional relationships tend to be more relationships between strangers than between intimates.[177] The combination of bureaucratization and technocratization can cause depersonalization and desensitization and, consequently, can have a dehumanizing effect. There is, therefore, a need to re-assert the humanitarian perspectives of both medicine and law. It might be that law can help in this respect in medicine and vice versa.

Further, there is a need to be sensitive not only to potentials for dehumanizing patients, but also to those which may dehumanize professionals dealing with patients and, in particular, psychiatrists. It has been proposed that some institutional environments, for instance those where administrators can override physicians, or where smooth running of the institution is seen as more important than maximizing therapy, or where the institution is organized in such a way that it insulates professionals from feelings of personal responsibility, can have a dehumanizing effect on medical staff working in them.[178] Such effects are of serious concern in relation to both physicians and the patients they treat.

Conflict of law and medicine

Sometimes the aims of medicine and law may be perceived as conflicting. This may occur insofar as law may be viewed as concentrating on rights, whereas medicine may be seen as concentrating on needs. Similarly, law functions primarily to recompense or avoid harm, while the primary aim of medicine is directed towards conferring benefit. Consequently, situations exist where the best of all worlds is not possible because these aims of avoiding harm and conferring benefit conflict.[179] As Gutheil *et al.* have stated, one must try to ensure that such conflicts do not leave a patient in a situation of having the worst of all worlds, in that neither his rights nor needs are respected.[180]

It is suggested that it may be useful to concentrate, first, on what law and medicine have to teach each other and, secondly, on some of their common, rather than conflicting, aims. For instance, whether one seeks to uphold rights or needs when these are in conflict, usually the most fundamental aim in both cases is that of the relief of suffering, whether that suffering is imposed because, for example, the patient's autonomy is not respected or because, in respecting his autonomy, his needs are not met.[181] By identifying such common aims a different resolution of the conflicts presented may be reached than would be the case if the starting point were, what is apparently, a totally adversarial position.

Medicine's influence on law

The discussion of the relationship of law and medicine has focussed, up to this point, principally on how law affects medicine. Medicine can also act directly to influence law. When it is questioned whose values and policies are being enacted as law, the possibilities are that those of individuals in the society, politicians, judges through courts, common interest groups such as physicians, institutions, society or the state, are being taken into account. The question becomes one of the power and influence of individuals or groups in terms of their ability to affect the enactment of legislation. In most western societies the medical profession, when it chooses to act, is a powerful political lobby. One current example of this, in England, is the alteration of the Police and Criminal Evidence Bill obtained by the British Medical Association. This alteration is to the effect that the confidentiality of medical records will be protected, because they will be excluded from the operation of the new legislative provisions which enable the police to have access to records to gather evidence.[182]

Further, it may be that we need to ask which values of any given decision-making participant should be enshrined in law, especially when there is conflict between the values of that participant. Obviously, there are no simple or universal answers, but in arriving at decisions as to which values are to be preferred in situations of conflict, theories such as Fried's on levels of decision-making may be helpful.[183] According to this theory, depending upon whether the decision-making relating to any given situation is at an individual, institutional or governmental level, the values which ought to be given priority may be different. For instance, the duty of 'personal care' and the values of individual integrity, faithfulness and trust would be overriding at a physician–patient level. On the contrary, utilitarian considerations, such as maximization of benefit, efficiency, etc., should not be taken into account at this level if they conflict with the physician's individual obligation of personal care to the patient. In contrast, these other values may predominate in decision-making at an institutional or governmental level.

Teaching medicine, law and ethics

Somewhat in contrast to law, medicine has tended to use an authoritarian model in teaching. Medical students, it is suggested, have been on the whole less well prepared than law students to deal with the paradox, uncertainty and conflict that practising a profession necessarily entails. This has been particularly true in relation to teaching the scientific elements of medicine (although this is now changing) and it may be for this reason that medical students often have difficulty in dealing with value conflicts.

It is well recognized that the half-life of knowledge is becoming shorter and shorter. Consequently, the aim in educating medical students should not be primarily to give them only the information which will suffice for a very short time, but rather to develop in them habits, and ways of thought, and a facility of gaining access to information, which will stand them in good stead throughout their professional lives. The aim is to create a desire and willingness and ability to learn and to continue learning. This is also true with respect to teaching medical students how to handle the ethical–legal–medical dilemmas that they will face in their future lives as professionals; students need to be given a framework or structure from which they can start to deal with such problems. It is no longer enough to think that these are simply personal value decisions and matters of intuition. To some degree, some of the changes in mental health legislation reflect and acknowledge these propositions.

Another important point is that it is not sufficient to teach one thing in theory and to do another in practice. It has been proposed that a very small 'group at the top' has the most influence on the ethical tone of an institution, perhaps as few as five people in an institution of a thousand employees.[184] Consequently, it is useless to sermonize to medical students about the need for ethics and proper values and legality of their conduct if, in practice, they perceive approaches inconsistent with what they have been taught. Practice is probably more influential in forming the attitudes of medical students than theory, particularly when that practice is carried out by people whom they respect and who are eminent in their particular fields of medicine, and whom students wish to emulate.

Professions and professionals
Trust and power

For reasons such as those discussed above, there has also been a lessening of trust in the professions in general, including the medical profession. It may also be that the greatly magnified power given to physicians and health care professionals by the new medical technology, and technology's potential not only for great benefit but also for serious harm, have caused both society itself and individual members of society who are subject to that power, to want to control it in some way and to a greater degree than in the past.

Conflict of values

It may also be that the perceived need to control professions and professionals arises from factors other than a desire to control the exercise of power. It has been proposed that there is an inherent duality and conflict between the two concurrent major underlying values of practitioners of medicine: those of self-interest and altruism.[185] Physicians may be personally vulnerable to this conflict and suffer as a result. Further, difficult decision-making situations may be created when there is either refusal to acknowledge the conflict or, even more so, when one motivation is confused with or promoted as the other. For instance, economic self-interest may be hidden by an altruistic façade when protection of the public is argued as the motivation for restricting medical licences or hospital privileges.[186] It may also be that self-interest is not involved, but conflict of interest still exists for a professional. To the extent that the professional sees himself or herself as an agent of society, and society's interest is in conflict with an individual patient's interest, this could be true. An area where this is particularly important in medicine in general is the allocation of scarce medical resources. There are even more precise examples involved in psychiatry, for example when the psychiatrist is seen as the agent of society who must protect society from danger caused by one of its members.

The nature of professional relationships

Professionals acting as the agents of society is one focus of the augmented general concern in many societies with civil libertarian issues. Both this focus and concern are relevant to medicine. There is less acceptance today, particularly among younger members of society, of paternalism on the part of health care professionals. There are many reasons for this, including: better general education, which means that the gap between the professional and the person he helps is lessened and a more egalitarian relationship results; the demystification of professions; perhaps, loss of status by some professions as they have become generally available as potential occupations for many members of developed western societies; the effect of consumerism, which causes professions to be seen as a product or service subject to the same rules and standards as other products or services;[187] less acceptance, in general, of authority, or at least of traditional authority, within the society; and more recognition of the uncertainty of professional decision-making.

This last factor may be one of the major thrusts towards changing both our educational system with respect to health care professions, and the way that those professionals treat persons who come to them for help. It is suggested that the change from the traditional authoritarian and paternalistic model of the physician–patient relationship to a more egalitarian one has been caused, in part, by the necessity to admit and articulate this uncertainty and communicate it to the patient. The doctrine of informed consent is one example of a legal requirement that would cause this phenomenon to occur.[188]

The nature of professions

Another issue which arises here is that of the nature of a profession, especially in terms of who owns or controls that profession. There are at least two opposing views.[189] The more socialistic approach is that a profession is owned by society; that society subsidizes the training of professionals and does so in order to benefit from their skills when trained; that society allows freedom of practice of a profession within certain limits, because this is the most beneficial situation for society; but that, essentially, a profession is held on trust by professionals to be used for the benefit of society. Pursuant to such a view, society retains the ultimate control of a profession and also the right to recall the 'legal ownership' of it from professionals when it feels that it needs to do so.[190] Such an approach enables a society to retain a large measure of control of professions and professionals.

An alternative view, and one which is more capitalistic and 'free enterprise', is that the professional, through his efforts in achieving professional status and, perhaps, even eminence, acquires a property right which he can then exploit for his own benefit. Pursuant to this approach society has a much less extensive right to regulate and interfere in the exercise of a profession. It is likely to be limited to doing so only when the professional's own exercise of his profession contravenes general concepts of public policy or public order and good morals. The current practice of

Canadian and American divorce courts of awarding one spouse who has helped the other to acquire professional training, a capitalized interest in that training, is one recognition of this approach to a profession.[191] While this trend is increasing, it may not be indicative of a general acceptance of professions as personal property. Rather, it may be simply an example of a legal device developed in order to do equity between two spouses. On the other hand, the use of such a device could have wider ramifications with respect to the view taken of the nature of professions by a society.

In conclusion, it may be that depending on the circumstances being dealt with, the choice between conflicting views of the nature of professions, discussed above, will differ. This could be regarded as an approach similar to that taken in situational ethics.[192] It is interesting to contemplate whether the law would accept such an approach, which would enable it to vary the basic concept it should use in any given circumstances.

Decision-making principles relevant to mental health legislation
Substantive and procedural rules
Law operates essentially via two types of rules: substantive rules and procedural rules. Both categories can operate as protective devices and in doing so, or in not doing so, reflect the values of a society. Substantive and procedural rules function differently but, usually, are designed to achieve the same overall aim. The relative degree of functioning of these rules *inter se* can vary with the stage of development of the issue to which they are being applied. When there is uncertainty about what substantive principle should be used, as there is in many areas where medicine and law interact, the primary safeguards used to govern decision-making may be procedural. It is hoped that by applying such procedures a proper decision outcome will be achieved in any given case. It should be noted that uncertainty necessitating the use of procedural safeguards can arise not only because of a lack of development of substantive principles, but also because the range of situations to which those principles should be applied can be so variable that it is not possible to predict in advance which principle is appropriate.

Balance in decision-making
There is a need to be aware constantly of the necessity to include a factor of balance in the decision-making concerning mental health care, whether that decision-making relates to formulation of laws, regulations for institutions, or issues concerning individual patients. This is the case

because there is no best of all worlds. There is usually no decision which is all good or benefit and no harm or risk; rather, there are competing harms and competing benefits. Sometimes it is said that there must be *compromise* to reach a decision result. While this is true, it is suggested that possibly this word should not be used. As already discussed, language is not neutral[193] and the word 'compromise' can have a connotation of 'selling out' some of the interests involved. Although it may be a euphemism, perhaps the word *balance* has a more desirable connotation. It also brings forward the idea of continually needing to re-assess and re-balance the issues involved. While on the subject of balance, it is worth noting the necessity to balance constructive and destructive criticism of a mental health system. Both can be effective means of achieving beneficial change when used in the right way and in the right places. Both can cause harm in some instances, although this is not intended. Further, it may not always be possible to identify in advance whether criticism will do good or cause harm. For instance, Mollica describes how the conflict which may arise in fighting for the humanization of mental health institutions, so that these institutions can provide adequate and effective care, can reveal the corrupt nature of these institutions and thus bring about their total destruction.[194] In contrast to unexpected conflict there may sometimes be unexpected agreement. Groups with different political ideologies may be promoting the same outcomes, but for different reasons. For instance, civil libertarians may be promoting rights of individual freedom and conservatives obligations of personal responsibility in similar attacks on certain provisions of a mental health care system.

Presumptions and decision-making
Initial presumptions

A factor which can reflect what are regarded as the more basic even among basic values, is the choice of initial presumption used to start a decision analysis. Sometimes these initial presumptions are unidentified. Although, in many cases, it may not make any difference in terms of decision outcome which of two opposing initial presumptions is used to commence a decision-making process, in border-line cases this may not be true.

It is worth querying whether legislation may be set up to look as though it is favouring one principle as an initial presumption (for example, autonomy) while its hidden agenda or the way in which it is able to be applied in practice may in fact favour another (for example, paternalism). One can speculate whether or not this is the case in theory, but to find out the true state of affairs empirical research would need to be carried out. Thus, for instance, when one compares the English and the Ontario mental health legislation, on paper the Ontario Act looks to be more protective of autonomy, and certainly has less paternalistically based exceptions to autonomy than the English Act.[195] What the final result is, in practice, depends not only on the written law, the legislation, but the social context in which it operates and the attitudes and behaviour of the professionals who apply it. Such professionals include not only those in health care but also, for instance, lawyers and courts who become involved because of alleged breaches of the legislation.

Presumptions and proof

Other presumptions which may be very important in relation to decision-making, and which also reflect value choices, are related to the burden of proof and standard of proof.

If one starts with an initial presumption of the liberty of the citizen, then the burden of proof should be on the person seeking to infringe this liberty. The standard of proof, if some of the more recent American authorities were to be followed, would be to the degree of 'clear and convincing evidence'.[196] This standard is something less than the usual criminal standard of proof 'beyond a reasonable doubt', and is more demanding than the usual private law standard of proof 'on the balance of probabilities'. The reason for adopting this standard is that when proof is not of past facts but relates to future predictions, as it does in establishing criteria for involuntary hospitalization, it is almost impossible to fulfil a standard of proof beyond a reasonable doubt. However, some courts in the United States have taken the view that proof on the balance of probabilities is an insufficiently demanding standard when it forms the basis on which a person's liberty is infringed.

It is worth noting that neither the English nor the Ontario Mental Health Act expressly provides for burden of proof or standard of proof. However, the general rule applied in statutory construction and relevant here, would be that he who alleges must prove and, consequently, the person alleging that the grounds for involuntary hospitalization are fulfilled would be the person who would have the burden of proving this. This approach can also be supported on the basis that the generally applicable rule is one of liberty and, therefore, any infringement of this liberty is an exception to the general rule and must be justified by the person relying upon the exception.

Conflict of interest

A further issue relevant to decision-making is the identification of any conflict of interest. For instance, this could be true of a third party decision-maker who is a member of the family of an incompetent person, or, even, some physicians. A physician could experience conflict of interest arising from many sources, including when he has a vested interest in ensuring that treatment is given. In one sense, the physician's desire to help, and if possible to cure the patient, means that he always has a vested interest. But something more than that is envisaged here. Such situations can include those as subtle as the physician having too great a personal identification with a certain treatment; alternatively they can be caused by the nature of medical training, which can sometimes tend to be overly interventionist, or does not sufficiently stress and deal with the fact that it is not always possible to cure. An example of a situation where there is more obvious conflict of interest for a physician is where he wishes to carry out medical research and his ability to do so hinges on the patient consenting to certain treatment.

Rules of construction

It is also worth mentioning a legal rule of construction in the current context. This rule requires that the general principle be given the widest operation and that exceptions to it be narrowly construed. As has been constantly reiterated throughout this paper, one of the basic and general principles of our society, and one which our law embodies, is that of freedom and liberty. Consequently, one could argue that statutes authorizing involuntary hospitalization, being exceptions to the rule protecting the liberty of persons, must be restrictively interpreted and not given any wider operation than their terms clearly encompass.

Role of psychiatrists in decision-making

Consideration of the proper role of the psychiatrist both in decision-making in medicine in particular and in society in general, is another important issue. The role played by psychiatrists reflects and creates values in mental health care, affects policy in this area, and often has many wider, more general ramifications.

It has been alleged that psychiatric consultation may be used to mask moral dilemmas arising in decision-making in medicine. 'Confusion has arisen in some professionals circles and in the public mind about the proper role of the psychiatrist in medicine and society. Being an expert in the science of human behaviour tends to be equated with knowing which behaviour is morally right. Psychiatrists are customarily called in to render opinions on what are, in fact, ethical and legal questions.'[197]

When one compares the English and Ontario mental health legislation, it would seem that under the English Act the role of the psychiatrist is more dominant in decision-making than under the Ontario Act. For instance, the scope of the patient's decision-making is wider and more protected under the Ontario Act.[198] Further, when the patient is incompetent to decide, or his decision is to be overridden, the persons who decide for him or who override his decision include persons other than psychiatrists under the Ontario Act, whereas in the English context the decision-making remains within the psychiatric profession.[199] This reflects a greater medicalization of the decision-making in England and probably indicates a more influential role for psychiatrists, not only in relation to these individual decisions but also in relation to the more general formulation of values and policies relevant to mental health care and, possibly, beyond this area.

When one turns to the area of psychiatrists' involvement in the criminal justice system, whether at the level of decision-making concerning responsibility, or conviction or sentencing of offenders, the issues become even more complex. Psychiatrists can view the influence which they exert regarding such decisions as either an unfair burden on them or a privilege, as within or without their proper area of expertise, and as being an appropriate or inappropriate function for a psychiatrist from an ethical point of view. However, whatever view one takes in these respects one point needs to be remembered: a judge does not have the liberty of refusing to make a decision. One consideration is, therefore, simply a relative one: that is, whether or not it is better to have a psychiatrist assisting the judge in some way in fulfilling this obligatory task.

CONCLUSION

Lawyers often speak of 'the seamless web of the common law'. The exploration of issues undertaken in this paper, although, of necessity, somewhat superficial, points to the wide and complex interrelationships of values, policy, psychiatry, ethics and law. These also constitute a 'seamless web': no single issue can be dealt with adequately without considering the multiple connections thrown up within this web. So complex is the area of interest canvassed by this paper that any attempt to draw broad conclusions risks producing generalities that are almost meaningless. There may, however, be one other general conclusion that is worth articulating.

It might be asked why we are so concerned about the rights of mentally ill people and with regulating in such minute detail and with such care and consideration our treatment of them, especially when most actors in this context have motives of at least doing no harm and usually of doing good.

There are many worse disasters in the world, perpetrated by people with evil motives, to which we could be turning our attention. And yet, it may be only by taking care in matters such as those raised in this paper and developing sensitivity to the issues involved, that ways of dealing with even larger problems will be found.

It is no accident that advances in medical science and medical situations are newsworthy and uniformly attract almost undivided attention from both the media and the general public. Everyone can relate in a personal way to a medical issue or problem. Consequently, the medical context could be the model for and forum in which approaches and controls that are needed in other areas of science, of seemingly even greater difficulty and impact, are recognized and developed. The most obvious of these areas is that of control of nuclear armaments.

I am deeply indebted to my research assistant, Ann Crawford, for her valuable contributions to this paper. Thanks are also due to Catherine Bry and Professor Michael Bridge for suggestions for stylistic changes.

NOTES

Abbreviations

The following abbreviations of Mental Health Acts are used throughout the notes:

MHA 1959 for Mental Health Act 1959, 7 & 8 Eliz. II c.75 (UK).

MH(A)A 1982 for Mental Health (Amendment) Act 1982 c.51 (UK).

MHA(O) for Mental Health Act, RSO 1980, c.262.

1. The same is true of the converse situation of psychiatry's involvement in law, as, for example, in criminal law.
2. See MHA 1959, ss.25 and 26, in each of which the 'safety' standard is enunciated. And see MH(A)A 1982, s.4 (2) (*b*), which enacts the requirement of 'treatability' of persons suffering from one of the minor disorders before they can be involuntarily hospitalized for treatment.
3. MH(A)A 1982, ss.12 (2) and 12 (3).
4. Mental Health Act, RSO 1980, c.269, s.8 (1) (*a*).
5. MHA(O), s.8 (1).
6. MHA(O), ss.9 and 14.
7. MH(A)A 1982, s.3 (1) (*b*).
8. For example, the Ontario legislation allows a maximum period of detention of 120 hours in the assessment phase; involuntary admission for treatment is a maximum of two weeks under the initial order (MHA(O), ss.9 and 14, respectively). Under the English legislation, short-term treatment is a maximum of 28 days, and long-term treatment is a maximum of six months pursuant to the initial order (MHA 1959, s.25 (4), and MH(A)A 1982, s.12 (2), respectively).

9. MH(A)A 1982, ss.41 and 3 (4) (*b*). See MHA 1959, s.3, for the establishment of Mental Health Review Tribunals.
10. MH(A)A 1982, s.40.
11. *X* v. *United Kingdom* [1982] 4 EHRR (1981 judgment).
12. MH(A)A 1982, s.28 (4) and Schedule 1.
13. MHA(O), s.31 (2) (*a*), which increases the number of times an application to a review board may be made.
14. Ibid., s.31 (4).
15. Ibid., s.33f (1) as enacted by s.67.
16. Ibid., s.35 (2).
17. Ibid., s.35 (4).
18. MH(A)A 1982 uses the term 'medical practitioner', which is defined in Medical Act 1956, 4 & 5 Eliz. II, c.76 (UK), s.7. The equivalent term in Ontario is 'physician', that is any registered medical practitioner. The term 'physician' in England tends to be reserved for a 'specialist physician', who, in Ontario, is often referred to as an 'internist'.
19. MH(A)A 1982, ss.44 (3) (*b*) and 44 (4). The medical practitioner is appointed for this purpose by the Secretary of State, and must consult two other persons who have been professionally concerned with the patient's medical treatment.
20. Ibid., s.48.
21. Ibid., s.49.
22. Ibid., s.16 (3).
23. Ibid., s.17.
24. Ibid., ss.29, 30 and 31. For a discussion of the purpose of these sections, see also 'Reform of Mental Health Legislation', paras. 49–51, Cmnd 8405 (1981) ('White Paper').
25. See MHA(O), ss.15 and 16, for provincial provisions. See also Criminal Code RSC 1970, c.C-34 (as amended), ss.465, 543 (2), 544 and 738 (5) and (6) for the federal provisions. M.E. Schiffer writes that the latter provisions 'provide ample opportunity for diversion at any stage of the trial process' (*Mental Disorder and the Criminal Trial Process*, Butterworths, Toronto, 1978, p.20).
26. MHA 1959, ss.60–64.
27. MH(A)A 1982, s.28 (4).
28. Constitution Act 1867, 30 & 31 Vict., c.3 (UK), s.91 (27).
29. Sections 545 (1) and 546 of the Criminal Code (note 25 above) are provisions giving to the Lieutenant Governor of a province the discretion to order hospitalization of persons found not guilty by reason of insanity and mentally disordered persons convicted and sentenced to incarceration in provincial prisons, respectively. Otherwise, no special sentences for mentally disordered offenders exist in the Criminal Code (see Schiffer, note 25 above, p. 227 and following, for a discussion of the possible ways in which the mentally disordered offender can be dealt with under Canadian law). It is interesting to note that Schiffer suggests that a uniform hospital order system should be adopted in the Criminal Code. This would bring the Canadian position more in line with the English one, although Schiffer rejects the features of the English system of indefinite renewal and orders for restricting discharge.
30. See Schiffer, Ch. 10, for a discussion of current law and practice regarding treatment and consent to treatment, with respect to the mentally disordered offender. See also M.A. Somerville, 'Refusal of treatment in "captive" circumstances', *Canadian Bar Review* (1985), forthcoming.
30a. MHA(O), s.13 (1).
30b. MHA(O), s.8 (1).
30c. This raises the issue of what constitutes a 'mental disorder' (see pp. 190–1, below) and that of 'rational' suicide.

31. It should be noted that the English Act demonstrates a recognition of this principle, in legislating provisions which contemplate previous and continuing social assessment of a patient in order to determine whether a service or method of providing for the person, other than involuntary hospitalization, exists (see the discussion on p. 158 above).

32. However, whether certain conduct is characterized as either conferring a benefit or avoiding harm, can be largely a question of semantics. Further, avoiding harm is, of course, a benefit. But what is envisaged here is that there are three positions. In a *negative* position, harm is inflicted or threatened. The avoidance of this harm or risk of harm would place a person in a *neutral* position. And a *positive* position is one in which the aim is to benefit the person.

33. See R. Anand, 'Involuntary civil commitment in Ontario: the need to curtail the abuses of psychiatry', *Canadian Bar Review*, 57 (1979), 250. See also F.R. Hartz, 'Dangerousness – postdict and predict: a review of the literature', *Legal Medical Quarterly*, 1–2 (1977–8), 204.

34. See below, p. 186.

35. D. Daube, 'Transplantation: acceptability of procedures and the required legal sanctions', in G.E.W. Wolstenhome and M. O'Connor (eds.) *Ethics in Medical Progress: with Special Reference to Transplantation* (London, J. & A. Churchill, 1966), p. 188.

36. M.A. Somerville, *Legal and Ethical Aspects of Decision-Making by and for Aged Persons in the Context of Psychiatric Care* (to be published by Nebraska Psychiatric Institute, University of Nebraska Medical Center).

37. G. Calabresi, *The Costs of Accidents* (New Haven and London, Yale University Press, 1970). See also below, pp. 185–6.

38. M.A. Somerville, 'Joinder of issue at the frontiers of biomedicine: a review essay on *Genetics, Ethics and the Law*, by George P. Smith, II' *University of New South Wales Law Journal*, 6 (1983), 103.

39. See above, pp. 159–61.

40. MHA 1959, s.47, and MH(A)A 1982, s.13 (1).

41. MHA 1959, s.48 (2).

42. MHA(O), s.28 (1).

43. It is interesting to note the very recent United States decision, *In re SL* 52 USLW 2074 (1983) (NJ Sup. Ct.), which held that patients in state mental hospitals who no longer meet state standards for civil commitment, but who nonetheless require some degree of custodial care may, under New Jersey law, remain confined pending efforts to place them in proper supportive settings outside an institution.

44. See below, pp. 81f, for a discussion of more general value and policy aspects of decision-making.

45. P.H. Wagner, 'North Carolina law and procedures regarding death and dying' (June 1983) *North Carolina Bar Association Foundation* II-3, citing *Durham Morning Herald*, 14 May 1983, pp. 11–15.

46. See, for example, Law Reform Commission of Canada Working Paper No. 24, 'Sterilization: implications for mentally retarded and mentally ill persons', Supply and Services Canada, Ottawa, 1979.

47. MH(A)A 1982, s.135 (1).

48. Ibid., s.136.

49. MHA(O), s.10 (1).

50. Ibid., s.11.

51. MHA 1959, s.27 (1). Further, one of the medical practitioners must be approved by the Secretary of State as having special experience in the diagnosis or treatment of mental disorder (MHA 1959, s.28 (2)).

52. MHA(O), s.9.
53. Ibid., s.14.
54. MH(A)A 1982, s.48.
55. Ibid.
56. MHA 1959, s.29 (3).
57. MHA(O), s.14 (4); MH(A)A 1982, s.12.
58. MHA(O), s.31; MH(A)A 1982, s.39.
59. C. Gilligan, 'New maps of development: new visions of maturity', *American Journal of Orthopsychiatry*, 52(2) (1982), 199. See also B. Bruteau, 'Neo-feminism and the next revolution in consciousness', *Cross Currents*, 27(2) (1977), 170.
60. Gilligan, ibid.
61. S. Toulmin, 'Equity and principles', *Osgoode Hall Law Journal*, 20(1) (1982), 1.
62. MH(A)A 1982, s.3 (4); MHA 1959, s.32 (4).
63. MHA(O), s.31.
64. See MH(A)A 1982, s.13 (1), for the nearest relative's right of discharge. See MHA 1959, s.48 (2), with respect to the barring certificate. It is interesting to note that the grounds on which the responsible medical officer may issue a barring certificate are that the patient, if discharged, would be likely to act in a manner dangerous to himself or others. This standard would appear to be more stringent than that required for admission (see above, pp. 159–61).
65. MHA 1959, s.48 (3).
66. MHA(O), s.31.
67. M.A. Somerville, *Consent to Medical Care* (Protection of Life Series, Law Reform Commission of Canada, Ottawa, 1979).
68. MH(A)A 1982, s.44 (1) (*b*); MHA(O), s.35 (2). See also below, p. 172, 'Categories of treatment'.
69. See below, pp. 183–5.
70. MH(A)A 1982, s.44 (1) (*b*).
71. See below, pp. 196–7.
72. See Dependent Adults Act, RSA 1980, c.D-32, and MHA(O). Section 1 (*g*) of the latter defines competence in terms of the function of being able to give informed consent.
73. MHA(O), s.1 (*g*).
73a. Somerville, note 30 above.
74. L.H. Roth, A. Meisl and C.W. Lidz, 'Tests of competency to consent to treatment', *American Journal of Psychiatry*, 134 (1977), 279.
75. Ibid.
76. Somerville, note 67 above.
77. M.A. Somerville, 'Structuring the issues in informed consent', *McGill Law Journal*, 26 (1981), 741.
78. The 'living will' is an example of such an approach. 'The living will' is a form letter, to be signed by adults, directing family and physicians in case of terminal illness to avoid heroic measures or extraordinary means of treatment, and to give palliative care and permit natural death.
79. B.L. Miller, 'Autonomy and Proxy Consent', *IRB*, 4(10) -1982), 1.
80. MH(A)A 1982, ss.43 (2) (*a*) and 44 (3) (*a*) and (*b*). These sections prohibit and allow, respectively, the administration of certain treatment if the patient is not 'capable of understanding the nature, purpose and likely effects of the treatment in question'.
81. MHA(O), s.1 (*g*): 'having the ability to understand the subject-matter in respect of which consent is requested and able to appreciate the consequences of giving or withholding consent'.

82. Mental Incompetency Act, RSO 1980, c.264, s.1 (*e*): 'such a condition of arrested or incomplete development of mind, whether ensuing from inherent causes or induced by disease or injury, or . . . suffering from such a disorder of the mind, that . . . care, supervision and control [is required] for . . . [the person's] protection and the protection of his property'. The Mental Incompetency Act legislates a wider definition of incompetency than the Mental Health Act (ibid.). The definition in the former Act is seemingly based more on the principle of beneficence than of autonomy. Incompetency is assessed mainly with reference to an objective judgment as to what is necessary for the person's protection. In comparison, the Mental Health Act definition requires a subjective analysis of the person's 'ability' to understand, and his 'appreciation' of consequences. The definition under the Mental Incompetency Act more closely represents the view that a rational decision outcome is required as an element of competency (see above, pp. 169–70).

83. This has been recommended by the Law Reform Commission of Canada with respect to findings of incompetency of persons on whom it is proposed to carry out sexual sterilization. See above, note 46.

84. MH(A)A 1982, ss.43, 44 and 49.

85. MHA(O), ss.35 (1) and 35 (2).

86. Ibid., s.35 (3).

87. Whether personal informed consent should be treated as a necessary, but not sufficient, condition for carrying out psychosurgery is a further issue. Not to allow competent persons to implement their freely taken decisions is also to restrict autonomy. However, concepts of 'public policy' and 'public order and good morals' regulate the acts to which consent may be given. See M.A. Somerville, 'Medical interventions and the criminal law: lawful or excusable wounding?', *McGill Law Journal*, 26 (1980), 82. It should also be noted that the doctrine of informed consent requires, as one of its elements, voluntariness. It should be questioned whether an involuntarily hospitalized patient is ever capable, simply because of the effect of his circumstances, of giving free and voluntary consent. But, such an approach although intended to be protective, could have the opposite effect. It may totally undermine the application of the doctrine of informed consent to institutionalized persons and result in them having less, rather than more, protection.

88. MH(A)A 1982, s.44, in particular s.44 (1) (*b*) for the 'three month' rule.

89. P.S. Appelbaum and T.G. Gutheil, 'Drug refusal: a study of psychiatric inpatients', *American Journal of Psychiatry*, 137 (1980), 3.

90. S.E. Many, 'Psychiatrists, state hospitals, and civil rights', *New York State Journal of Medicine*, 80 (1980), 1873 on 1874.

91. Ibid.

92. MH(A)A 1982, ss.44 (1) (*a*) and 44 (5).

93. See L. Gostin, 'A review of the Mental Health (Amendment) Act. III. The legal position of patients while in hospital', *New Law Journal*, 132 (1982), 1199, where he states that electroconvulsive therapy is likely to be included in regulations concerning treatment requiring consent or a second opinion under MH(A)A 1982, s.44.

94. See Calabresi, note 37 above.

95. MH(A)A 1982, s.49.

96. See forthcoming Working Paper of the Law Reform Commission of Canada, 'Psychosurgery and behaviour modification'.

97. J.G. Fleming, *The Law of Torts*, 6th edn (The Law Book Company Ltd, Nettey, South Australia, 1983) pp. 146–53.

98. Ibid., pp. 30–2.
99. R.B. Sklar, *Aversive Conditioning and the Mentally Retarded* (Faculty of Law, McGill University, forthcoming publication).
100. See, for example, *Board of Governors of Seneca College of Applied Arts and Technology* v. *Bhadauria* (1983) 124 DLR (3d) 193 (SCC).
101. For more detailed discussion of the torts referred to here see Fleming, note 98 above, pp. 23–30 and 97–100.
102. *Tarasoff* v. *Regents of University of California* (1976) 551 P. 2d 384 (Supreme Court of California).
103. See, for example, Criminal Code, note 25 above, at s.202 (1).
104. For a discussion by a court of these issues, see *Helling* v. *Carey* (1974) 83 Wash. 2d 514 (Supreme Court of Washington en banc).
105. MHA 1959, s.26, as amended by MH(A)A 1982, s.4 (2). See also note 161 below.
106. MH(A)A 1982, s.4 (1) (*b*).
107. At the time the 1959 Act was promulgated twenty-one years was the age of majority.
108. MHA 1959, s.4 (1): 'mental illness, *arrested or incomplete development of the mind*, psychopathic disorder, and *any other disorder or disability of the mind*' (emphasis added).
109. 'Reform of Mental Health Legislation', note 24 above, paras. 8–10. However, it is not made clear which provisions are meant to be applicable to the mentally handicapped, particularly given that the White Paper had contemplated the use of the term 'mental handicap' instead of 'mental impairment' as was used in the Act (MH(A)A 1982, s.1 (2)). Gostin, (note 94 above) suggests that it is mainly those provisions which merely require 'mental disorder' which will be applicable to the mentally handicapped.
110. MH(A)A 1982, ss.1 (2) and 26 (2) (*a*).
111. MHA(O), s.1 (*f*).
112. *Clark* v. *Clark* (1983), 40 OR (2d) 383, (Provincial County Court).
113. In some jurisdictions, guardianship orders are referred to as 'commitment orders', in which case these orders must be distinguished from involuntary hospitalization procedures, which are sometimes referred to as 'involuntary civil commitment'.
114. Note, in this respect, that MHA 1959, ss.33 and 34, as amended by MH(A)A 1982, ss.7 and 8, could itself provide for a limited system of guardianship for '[a] very small number of mentally disordered people who do not require treatment in hospital either informally or formally, nevertheless need close supervision and some control in the community as a consequence of their mental disorder' ('Reform of Mental Health Legislation', note 24 above, paras. 43–5).
115. See note 72 above.
116. Mental Health Act, RSA 1980, c.M-13.
117. Letter to the author from Joel Christie, Public Guardian of Alberta, 28 March 1983.
118. MH(A)A 1982, s.44 (3) (*b*).
119. MHA(O), s.35 (2).
120. Although the next-of-kin is usually the decision-maker for an incompetent adult patient, there is some doubt whether this is actually authorized by common law – that is, whether it is authorized in situations where it is not provided by statute that next-of-kin may act as such decision-maker.
120a. See Somerville, note 30 above.
121. *Regina* v, *Ogg-Moss* (1981) 5 Leg. Med. Q. 146 (C.A. Ont.).

122. Criminal Code, note 25 above, s.43.
122a. *Ogg-Moss* v. *R*, Supreme Court of Canada, October 1984 (unreported; to be reported in Dominion Law Reports).
123. Editorial, 'The right to die', *The Lancet*, I (1983), 1197.
124. MH(A)A 1982, s.56.
125. Ibid., s.53.
126. MH(A)A 1982, parts II and III.
127. Criminal Code, note 25 above.
128. See below, p. 204.
129. See Schiffer, note 25 above.
130. MHA 1959, s.65, as amended by MH(A)A 1982, s.28 (1).
131. Criminal Code, note 25 above, ss.545 and 546.
132. For instance, a person held pursuant to a 'hospital order' under the English Act, has reduced rights as compared with a civilly committed patient. For example, he has more limited access to a Mental Health Review Tribunal and his nearest relative cannot apply for his discharge.
133. Personal communication, Orville Endicott, President, Canadian Association for the Mentally Retarded, Toronto, regarding the Emerson Bonner case in New Brunswick.
134. Personal communication, G. Sharpe, legal advisor to the Ontario Ministry of Health, Toronto; W. McCalla, Solicitor-General's Department, Ottawa.
135. MH(A)A 1982, s.19, incorporates this approach by providing that a court cannot make a hospital order with respect to a person suffering from a psychopathic disorder or mental handicap unless there is medical evidence that medical treatment in hospital is likely to alleviate or prevent a deterioration in the offender's condition.
136. *Jones* v. *United States*, 52 USLW 5041 (United States Supreme Court 1983).
137. See Somerville, note 67 above.
138. *Commissioner of Correction* v. *Myers*, 399 N.E. 2d 452 (Sup. Jud. Ct. Mass. 1979).
139. G.J. Annas, 'Prison hunger strikes: why the motive matters', *The Hastings Center Report*, 12(6) (1982), 21; Somerville, note 30 above.
140. *Attorney General of British Columbia* v. *Astaroff* [1983] 6 W.W.R. 332 (B.C.S.C.); (1983) 10 W.C.B. 223 (B.C.C.A.); (1983) 6 C.C.C., 3d 498 (S.C. and C.A.).
141. K.C. Micetich, P.H. Steinecker and D.C. Thomasma, 'Are intravenous fluids morally required for a dying patient?', *Archives of Internal Medicine*, 143 (1983), 975.
142. See below, pp. 187–8.
143. See Calabresi, note 37 above.
144. Editorial, 'Ethics and the nephrologist', *The Lancet*, I (1981), 594. See also M.A. Somerville, Letter to the Editor re 'Ethics and the nephrologist', *The Lancet*, I (1981), 1109.
145. See Part I above.
146. C.J. Smith, 'Innovation in mental health policy: the political economy of the community mental health movement 1965–1980', unpublished paper presented at 'Community Mental Health Care in Crisis', Association of American Geographers Meeting, Denver, Colorado, April 1983.
147. J.F. Fletcher, *Moral Responsibility: Situation Ethics at Work* (Philadelphia, Westminster Press, 1967).
148. See above, pp. 159–63.
149. MH(A)A 1982, s.44 (1) (*b*).
150. R. Fein, 'What is wrong with the language of medicine?', *New England Journal of Medicine*, 306 (1982), 863.

151. M.A. Somerville, 'Birth technology, parenting and "Deviance"', *International Journal of Law and Psychiatry*, 5(2) (1982), 123.
152. MHA(O), s.29.
153. MH(A)A 1982, s.57.
154. Ibid., s.58.
155. Ibid., s.52; MHA(O), s.20.
156. Smith, note 147 above.
157. P.K. Bridges, Review of M. O'Callaghan and D. Carroll, *Psychosurgery: A Scientific Analysis* (1982), *The Lancet*, I (1983), 962.
158. MH(A)A 1982, s.16 (3).
159. Gostin, note 94 above, p. 1130.
160. See MH(A)A 1982, ss.1 (2) and 2 (1). These sections do not use the terms minor or major disorders, but these were suggested by Gostin in part I of his article (ibid.).
161. See, for example, MH(A)A 1982, s.4 (2).
162. See, for example, in Quebec, An Act Respecting Health Services and Social Services, RSO 1977, c.S-5, s.4. It could be argued that it is a fundamental human right to have access to a basic level of health care, or at least to that level reasonably available in any given society. In this case, rights to health care would exist in all societies, regardless of the nature of their health care systems or whether statutory rights to health care had been enacted.
163. D.J. Hunter, 'The privatisation of public provision', *The Lancet*, I (1983), 1264 at 1267.
164. See above, p. 190.
165. Code pénal, art. 63 (2).
166. P. Lombard, P. Macaigne and B. Oudin, *Le médecin devant ses juges* (Paris, Robert Laffont, 1973), Chapter 1.
167. See Micetich *et al.*, note 142 above.
168. Smith, note 147 above, at p. 15.
169. It should be noted that it is not being suggested here that ends necessarily justify means.
170. Smith, note 147 above, at pp. 15–16.
171. Ibid., p. 15.
172. Ibid.
173. R.M. Ratzan, 'Cautiousness, risk, and informed consent in clinical geriatrics', *Clinical Research*, 30 (1982), 345.
174. See Somerville, note 36 above. See also below, p. 201 and following.
175. *Mount Isa Mines* v. *Pusey* (1970) 125 CLR 383, 395 (Windeyer J., High Court of Australia).
176. See below, pp. 199–201.
177. See, for example, R.A. Burt, *Taking Care of Strangers: The Rule of Law in Doctor–Patient Relations* (New York, Free Press, 1979).
178. Many, note 91 above.
179. M.A. Somerville, *The Law and Mental Health Care for Competent and Incompetent Elderly Persons*, forthcoming publication in *Disturbed Behaviour in the Elderly* (New York, S.P. Medical and Scientific Books, 1983).
180. T.G. Gutheil, H. Bursztajn, A. Kaplan, R. Hamm and A. Brodsky, 'The psychiatrist as guardian *ad litem*: the team approach to cases of suspected incompetence', 6 April 1983 (unpublished).
181. M.A. Somerville, 'Pain and suffering at interfaces of medicine and law' (forthcoming publication).
182. See R. Deitch, 'The Police and Criminal Evidence Bill', *The Lancet*, I (1983), 942. There is no intention, here, to imply that such an amendment is not desirable. Rather, the purpose is to note it and how it was achieved.

183. C. Fried, *Medical Experimentation: Personal Integrity and Social Policy* Amsterdam, North-Holland Publishing Co., 1974).

184. B. Barber, J. Lilly, J.L. Makarushka and D. Sullivan, *Research on Human Subjects (A Problem of Social Control in Medical Experimentation)* (New York, Russell Sage Foundation, 1973).

185. A. Jonsen, 'Sounding board – watching the doctor', *New England Journal of Medicine*, 308 (1983), 1531.

186. It should be noted that it is not being suggested that licensing is not in the public interest, simply that this may not always be the real motive for promoting it. Obviously, there are many situations of mixed motivation and some in which both altruism and self-interest will indicate the same decision outcome. The point is that when they do not, care must be taken to distinguish between them in order to determine what the decision should be.

187. This could be caused, in part, by professionals being perceived as selling their professional skills primarily on the basis of maximizing their income. This may be acceptable in some professions, but usually causes adverse reactions when it occurs in the health care professions. Again, it is not suggested that health care professionals should not try to maximize their income. Rather, this cannot be a primary, or at least overt, aim.

188. See Somerville, note 67 above. See also Somerville, note 77 above.

189. P.F. Camenisch, 'Commentary: on the professions', *The Hastings Center Report*, 6(5) (1976), 8.

190. The legal concept of a trust involves conceptualizing two notional, proprietary interests in any given piece of property. The property may be physical or non-physical (incorporeal). The true owner holds what is called the equitable interest in the property (thus society is the equitable owner of the professions), while the apparent owner, who holds the property on trust for the true owner, is regarded as holding the legal interest (the professional is the legal owner of the profession). The person with the equitable interest can recall the legal interest, giving him the totality of interests in, that is full ownership of, the property.

191. See K. Connell-Thouez, 'Matrimonial property regimes in Quebec before and after the reform of 1981: adapting traditional institutions to modern reality', in K. Connell-Thouez and B. Knoppers (eds.) *Contemporary Trends in Canadian Family Law* (Toronto, Carswell, 1984).

192. Above, pp. 187–8.

193. See above, p. 189 and note 151.

194. R.F. Mollica, 'From asylum to community: the threatened disintegration of public psychiatry', *New England Journal of Medicine*, 308 (1983), 367.

195. Part I above.

196. *State of Texas* v. *Addington* (1980) 588 S.W. 2d 569.

197. M. Perl and E.E. Shelp, 'Psychiatric consultation, masking moral dilemmas in medicine', *New England Journal of Medicine*, 307 (1982), 618, 620.

198. See above, pp. 167–8 and 172–5.

199. See above, p. 158.

The Danish experience: one model of psychiatric testimony to courts of law

VILLARS LUNN

The theme of my paper, experiences in respect of psychiatric testimony to courts of law, is obviously wide-ranging and of general forensic importance, which necessitates a rather restricted delimitation. So, on the basis of experiences from my own country, Denmark, I have chosen to subdivide the subject as follows:

1. To describe the general lines laid down by the Director of Public Prosecutions to help characterise those categories of psychically anomalous offenders in which the question of applying special measures or sanctions might arise.

2. With the provisions of the Danish Penal Code as the starting point, I shall discuss the psychiatric criteria which must be fulfilled before sanctions, alternative to punishment, are considered applicable.

3. Finally I shall review the actual procedure or practice in Denmark as regards the production of psychiatric testimony in court.

Historical background
By way of introduction, however, a short historical outline might be useful. Considering the small size of my country this might sound pretentious, but it is my impression – and thereby my justification – that the developments in Denmark within this field might be regarded as representative of the developments in the western world as a whole.

In 1930 the Danish Penal Code was fundamentally revised, particularly as regards the provisions dealing with psychically anomalous offenders. This revision came at a time characterized by great optimism and confidence regarding the effect of psychological and psychiatric treatment as opposed to punishment, treatment being considered the most appropriate sanction for preventing criminal relapse. The ideology of treatment represented the prevailing opinion at this time among not only forensic psychiatrists, but quite a number of progressive jurists as well.

The product of this way of thinking was the introduction of a multitude of sanctions or provisions as alternatives to punishment. Foremost of these, and given as a matter of course, was real psychiatric treatment, whether in an outpatient setting or after removal of the individual to a psychiatric hospital or institution for mental defectives. Additional options were placement in preventive detention, in a special remand home for psychopaths, an institution for juvenile delinquents, or a home for inebriates. The crucial point, the common denominator of all these measures, is that they are in the main not time-limited, the idea being that the suspension or cancellation of the sanctions should be determined primarily by the outcome of treatment, regardless of the seriousness of the crime.

In the nineteen thirties and forties the ideology of treatment sailed downwind. First of all the special remand homes were extensively used as a sanction not only for crimes of violence and other serious crimes, but increasingly for more commonplace kinds of criminality, such as simple unlawful gains, as well.

As was to be expected, this development engendered its reaction during the fifties and sixties: the ideology of treatment met with growing scepticism, to begin with among jurists and the general population, but gradually among psychiatrists as well. The reasons or justifications for this anti-treatment attitude were above all an animosity towards the concept of time unlimited sanctions as such. But also the disproportion in some cases between a trivial offence and the resulting long detention was increasingly criticized. Last, but not least, the empirical evaluation of the appropriateness of these special measures in respect of preventing criminal relapse showed them to be disappointing or at best dubious.

The result of this development was rather dramatic: in 1973 the Danish Penal Code underwent a revision, the implied result of which was that all special sanctions or provisions alternative to punishment were abolished – apart from sentence to real psychiatric treatment, either as an outpatient or after confinement to hospital or institution for mental defectives. It is noteworthy that this amendment implied an abolition of the well-known special remand hospital for psychopaths in Herstedvester. In 1975 the principal paragraphs concerning the legal status of psychically anomalous offenders – psychotic as well as non-psychotic – were reformulated in accordance with the ideological development just described.

As the last step in this development it might be mentioned that the pendulum in the last few years has once again shown a tendency to swing in the opposite direction. Thus, the number of offenders subjected to psychological and psychiatric observation in the early eighties once more shows a rising trend, following a steep fall in the seventies. Coincident with this possible revival in Denmark of the psychological viewpoint in forensic psychiatry, however, the ideology of 'equal rights' or 'normalization' for mentally abnormal offenders is much discussed, especially in terms of the claim for the 'right to punishment' of unmistakably psychotic patients.

As mentioned above, my justification for presenting this short historical survey has been the notion that the development described might be paradigmatic for a more general change of attitude regarding the concepts of crime and punishment. Legal philosophers talk of it in terms of neo-classicism in the law of procedure, which involves minimizing or ignoring individual psychopathological traits and applying instead a 'fixed-rate principle', characterized by a direct proportionality between the seriousness of the crime and the gravity of the sanction, irrespective of the personality in question.

Categories of offenders warranting psychiatric observation

According to the Danish Administration of Justice Act, psychiatric observation is indicated:

1. If there is a presumption that the accused or the defendant is insane (psychotic) or mentally deficient.
2. If incidentally (say, on account of the nature of the criminal offence) there might be a presumption that the defendant's mental condition is abnormal to such a degree that special measures alternative to punishment might be brought into play.
3. If the charge concerns a felony such as manslaughter, arson with no economic gain, or gross sexual offence.
4. If special categories of alcoholism and drug addiction are dealt with, or if the offender is more than 60 years old and charged with a crime for the first time.

Psychiatric criteria for exemption from punishment

I shall now outline the Danish viewpoint and measures concerning the following spheres within forensic psychiatry:

1. The provisions for dealing with those psychically abnormal offenders who, according to Scandinavian criminal law, are absolutely and unconditionally exempted from punishment.
2. The provisions for dealing with those who are relatively or conditionally exempted from punishment.

Because of the close affinity of the Scandinavian societies socially and culturally, and thus also as far as fundamental legal points of view are concerned, an explanation of conditions in Denmark will in general also cover the conditions in Norway and Sweden.

Regarding point 1 above, paragraph 44 of the *Norwegian* Criminal Code states:

> Acts committed by persons who are insane or unconscious at the time of committing the act are not punishable.

The corresponding section of the *Danish* Code (paragraph 16) says (in close accordance with the Swedish Code):

> 1. Acts committed by persons irresponsible owing to insanity or similar conditions or pronounced mental deficiency are not punishable.
> 2. If, however, the psychotic state is caused by intake of alcohol or similar intoxicants, punishment – under special circumstances – may be used.

As will be seen, we are with these two wordings in the centre of the discussion that has been carried on since Samuel Pufendorf's classical work *Elementorum jurisprudentiae naturalis libri* (1660), on the question of the responsibility of psychically abnormal persons and the criteria of exemption from punishment. Four fundamentally different principles or views can be distinguished:

1. The purely biological or medical criterion.
2. The psychological criterion, also called the metaphysical criterion.
3. A mixed or combined medicopsychological criterion.
4. The so-called penitential criterion which involves the question of the offender being susceptible to punishment.

In Norwegian criminal law the *biological criterion* has found expression. Here the law has accepted that exemption from punishment is automatically connected with establishment of insanity at the time of committing the punishable act. In other words, in this connection the metaphysical concept of responsibility versus irresponsibility has been definitively eliminated in Norwegian legislation, for if the court decides, on the basis of the experts' findings, that the offender was insane or unconscious at the time of committing the punishable act, then he must be found not guilty, irrespective of whether there is any relation between his insanity and the act with which he is charged. On this principle the experts' task is fairly simple, for they only have to establish, once the necessary examinations have been made, whether any of the psychical abnormalities mentioned in the Criminal Code existed at the time of committing the act. It is no concern of the experts to state whether there was any connection between the offender's mental state and the punishable act; whether there is any reason to suppose that because of his mental state he has had no insight into or been unable to realize the nature of the act, its unlawfulness or criminality; whether there is any reason to suppose that he had no control of himself and no faculty of normal motivation; and finally, whether there is reason to suppose that he would be susceptible to punishment or not. The experts will expressly *not* have to make any statement in these respects.

The reason for adopting this strictly biological criterion – which many people will undoubtedly find radical and provocative – lies in a rejection in principle of the concept of partial insanity. The point of view is that it is impossible in any case of psychosis to decide where the disease ends and where normal thinking begins. The possibility is thus rejected of a psychotic state of mind being able to act 'partially' in certain cases – that is, leaving certain 'parts' of the mind untouched. It is supposed that the psychopathological mechanisms influence all of the defendant's motivations and actions, and consequently that it is unjustifiable to make provisions for a criminal act independent of the insanity.

I must declare myself in principle a follower of this logical medical criterion, which from a psychiatric point of view must seem rational as well as realistic. Later, during my explanation of Danish legislation, I shall revert to this matter, but first I will make some comments on the administrative consequences of introducing the biological criterion in Norway.

It has been maintained, with some justice, that the adoption of this principle in fact means that it is the psychiatric experts who decide whether a defendant shall be found guilty or not. It is true that the court can in theory decide whether or not it will accept the experts' evaluation of the mental state of the defendant. But in fact the judges, who must in this respect consider themselves laymen, will generally feel bound by the experts' evaluation. A heavy responsibility is therefore imposed on the experts because the law, when formulated on the basis of a merely medical criterion, forces them to pronounce with the highest degree of certainty (the law does not allow any doubt) on a concept of insanity which has no exact criteria and very uncertain limits. In consequence of this categorical request it has become legal usage in Norway for a defendant to be found insane only if it can virtually *be proved* – through the demonstration of indisputable, positive symptoms – that he was in a psychotic state of mind at the time of committing the act.

It is quite clear that this request for a simple and unambiguous delimitation must result in a corresponding reduction or narrowing of the concept of insanity, and it cannot be denied that this will lead to a conflict with the usual tendency in modern clinical psychiatry; in fact, it means that a number of paranoid states developed on a characterological basis, such as jealousy and querulous paranoia, must be excluded from the insanity paragraph although from a psychological point of view there is a clear connection between the mental abnormality and the criminal act. However, this consequence of the biological criterion is less alarming in that other legal provisions open a possibility of sentencing such psychically anomalous persons to custody – a form of sanction used, of course, on most of the offenders found not guilty under the insanity paragraph.

In contrast to the biological or medical criterion, the *psychological criterion* attaches decisive importance to the responsibility concept. According to this principle, insanity is *not* considered exonerating but importance is attached to the question of whether the defendant did or did not understand that he was acting contrary to the law. The implications of this criterion are familiar from the M'Naghten Rules, and I shall therefore not go into details, but merely point out that according to Scandinavian thinking the psychological or metaphysical criterion is based on a fundamental failure to appreciate the global nature of psychopathological mechanisms; accordingly, the experts in psychiatry are facing a theoretically insoluble problem and in consequence the criterion is, and has been for a long time, considered obsolete.

This said, I must, much to my regret, admit that Danish legislation on insane offenders is still built on a mixture of *medical and psychological criteria*. As mentioned above, the Danish Criminal Code (paragraph 16) says that acts committed by persons irresponsible owing to insanity or similar conditions or pronounced mental deficiency are not punishable. Thus the metaphysical concept of responsibility remains! Seen against the background of what I have just said this may sound like a *contradictio in adjectio*. The fact is, however, that according to Danish legal usage related to the paragraph on insanity, psychiatrists are distinctly not meant to state their opinion on the question of responsibility. As in Norway, the task of the forensic psychiatrist in this respect is purely diagnostic, since he is required to state only whether at the time of the crime the offender can be supposed to have been insane or not, or whether he is markedly mentally deficient. As far as the medical statement is concerned, Danish legislation on the legal status of the insane is thus based on the biological criterion.

Why then has the concept of responsibility been retained in the text of the law? There are two reasons. First, jurists want to emphasize that the question of culpability should not be primarily a medical decision. This would be the case if exemption from punishment depended on the diagnosis, since in reality the court has no way of verifying the latter. In the last instance the decision has to be placed in the hands of the judge and this is possible only if he can reserve the right to decide whether the abnormal state diagnosed by the expert should exempt from punishment. Therefore the word 'irresponsible' has been inserted in the text of the Danish Code rather as a buffer between the medicobiological and the legal point of view.

Second, maintenance of the concept of responsibility implies an admission of the fact that in certain cases it may seem doctrinaire and rigid to stick consistently to the biological criterion. Particularly in the case of certain paranoid forms of insanity, offences may occur where a psychological connection with the mental disorder is rather unlikely. If, for instance, during the development of a mental disease, a habitual thief continues to steal, it would seem somewhat unnatural suddenly to put the blame on his mental disorder. Likewise persons with pronounced but less severe mental disease are not uncommonly able to look after their business in an intelligent and responsible way, and it would seem unreasonable not to hold them responsible if for mere profit they started swindling. In any case it is understandably difficult to convince the jurists of this.

Danish legislation on the culpability of the insane is therefore a compromise between medical and legal views. I find this a disadvantage because in my opinion the consistent application of the biological criterion, as adopted in Norwegian legislation, is the only valid standpoint from a psychiatric point of view. I consider it a good thing, however, that according to Danish legal usage psychiatrists are exempted from including the concept of responsibility in their expert opinion, just as I must admit that it is very exceptional for a judge to find an offender responsible and consequently liable to punishment if the psychiatric experts have declared him insane or markedly mentally deficient. All things considered, I would say (again from a psychiatric point of view) that Scandinavian legislation is satisfactory and uncontroversial as far as psychotic offenders – in the proper sense of the word – are concerned.

Far more complicated and controversial are the problems attached to the legal status of non-psychotic but nevertheless mentally abnormal offenders. Regarding this heterogeneous group of mentally deviant persons, section 69 of the Danish Criminal Code says:

> If, at the time of committing the punishable act, the psychic condition of the perpetrator involved defective development, or impairment or disturbance of the psychic functions of a nature other than that indicated in section 16 of this Act, and if special

measures may be considered more expedient for preventing criminal relapse, the Court can decree the application of such measures (in accordance with section 68 of the Criminal Code).

Among those conditions characterized in the Code by the words 'defective development, impairment or disturbance of the psychic functions' some categories of moderate mental deficiency and psychopathy are obviously the most important. To these must be added cases of narcomania with obvious psychopathological background or consequences, special categories of chronic alcoholism, and certain states of senility (the last particularly in relation to indecent acts of the senile towards children). Finally a group of anomalous sexual offenders, for instance exhibitionists and a heterogeneous group of borderline cases, might be embraced by section 69 of the Criminal Code.

In cases such as those mentioned here, the court, supported by psychiatric opinion, has to decide whether special measures such as psychiatric treatment must be considered more expedient for preventing criminal relapse than punishment. If detention in a psychiatric hospital is found necessary, the court, in accordance with the law, will as a rule fix a time limit of one year (section 68). In contrast, offenders who are exempted from punishment pursuant to section 16 – that is to say, psychotic patients or severe mental defectives – will be sentenced to time-unlimited measures.

Concerning the so-called section 69 cases the court is, as mentioned previously, confronted with two possibilities: either to decree ordinary punishment or to decree application of special measures according to section 68 of the Criminal Code. It is thus a question of 'either/or'. From this it follows that the third possibility – namely a reduced or milder sentence – is ignored in Scandinavian legislation. In the case of persons with 'impairment or disturbance of the psychic functions', reduction of punishment is looked upon as an antiquated retributive measure that should not exist in rational criminal legislation, the sole purpose of which must be the protection of society. There is, however, one exception to this rule: If the punishable act has been committed in a state of intense agitation or other transitory unbalance of the mind, the punishment must be reduced. To decide whether and to what degree such a state of transitory mental unbalance has been present is one of the most difficult tasks with which the forensic psychiatrist is confronted.

Regarding the decision of whether to impose ordinary punishment or special measures, it must be noted finally that the general attitude of the courts now tends increasingly towards punishment and away from treatment or detention in hospital. One has to realize that this attitude, being an expression of the ideology of 'normalization', will dominate the legal usage for a number of years yet.

The Danish Medico-Legal Council

The next topic I would like to discuss is purely technical: namely, the way in which cooperation between courts and psychiatric experts is organized. While the subject may appear to be without actual psychiatric interest, the following are undeniably problems which forensic psychiatrists cannot neglect:

1. The role of expert witnesses in trials.
2. The objective value of cross-examinations.
3. The importance of establishing uniform procedures and common guidelines within all jurisdictions.
4. The question of the absolute objectivity and independence of experts.

Denmark has had for more than 70 years a system which, in our opinion, has rationally solved a number of these problems. The history of the Danish Medico-Legal Council goes back about 300 years. Around 1650 the King ordered the members of the Faculty of Medicine to appear as expert witnesses in cases involving medical problems. Later, this function was taken over by the so-called Royal Health Board, which until 1909 discharged these consultative responsibilities in legal cases and was the administrative authority in all matters pertaining to health. By an Act of 1909 the Royal Health Board was divided into a governmental department, the National Health Service, which is a purely administrative department, and the Medico-Legal Council, a consultative medical board quite independent of the health administration. In 1935 a special Act was passed defining the functions of the Council. Its tasks are to give such medical and pharmaceutical opinions as are decisive for the legal relationships of individuals. These opinions can be asked for only by the courts and public authorities, not by private persons. Solicitors and, in criminal cases, counsel for the defence can ask for the opinion of the Council via the court, the county or the prosecutor.

The Medico-Legal Council consists of 35 medical experts covering all the fields of medicine, including the work of the general practitioner and pharmacist. Eleven of the 35 experts are ordinary members. They constitute the main body of the Council, and at least two of them must give an opinion in each case enquired into by the Council. These 11 members comprise one specialist in internal medicine, one in surgery, one in obstetrics and gynaecology, one in forensic medicine and seven psychiatrists. The remaining 24 experts are extraordinary members, among whom one or several are summoned to participate instead of one of the permanent members of the Council or together with these when the nature of a case renders it necessary. Both the ordinary members, who are appointed under the Royal Seal, and the extraordinary members, who are appointed by the Ministry of Justice, are appointed for a term of 6 years upon the recommendation of the members of the Council. Both groups of members must be active in their special field, their Council function being thus a part-time function only. Finally one or two members of the legal profession (jurists) are attached to the Council. They examine all cases, offer guidance to the medical experts concerning legal problems, and attend to the clerical work. The legal experts act in a purely advisory capacity and never give opinions.

It must be emphasized that the fees of members of Council are paid from public funds (the Ministry of Justice), the permanent members being paid annually and the consultant extraordinary members receiving their fees for individual cases. The opinions given are free of charge, and it is obvious that the position of the institution as an independent adviser is strengthened by the fact that there is no question of money between the Council and the parties involved. Consequently, the appearance of doctors as expert witnesses in court in Denmark is necessary only in extremely rare cases, since the authoritative opinion of the Medico-Legal Council is normally considered the most effective evidence.

In the vast majority of cases the opinion of the Council is given solely on the basis of the medical certificates, hospital records and autopsy reports available in the case, but the Council has the opportunity to make a direct study of any macroscopic or microscopic specimen and to examine the person, possibly by admitting him to a member's hospital department.

Generally, the cases must be enquired into by three members at least. In most cases the individual members express their opinions in writing, but if the nature of the case renders it necessary, meetings are held, presided over by the President, where direct discussions take place. Negotiations may be conducted with any member of the medical profession who has knowledge of the person or the case in which the Council has to give its opinion, and such negotiations are compulsory in certain cases when the attitude of the Council differs essentially from the reports at hand.

The proceedings of the Council are published as a special official notice. As a rule, its opinions of the Council must be substantiated by arguments, particularly when the Council disagrees with a medical report given in the case.

The members cannot be examined by the court, but prior to the trial of a case the court, counsel for the prosecution and counsel for the defence

Table 1. *Cases enquired into by the Danish Medico-Legal Council in 1981*

Category	Number	Percentage
Psychiatric cases	988	38
Intoxicated drivers	820	31
Disputed paternity	382	14
Medico-legal cases (malpractice etc.)	277	11
Cases concerning drug-misuse	119	5
Administrative cases	40	1
Total	2626	100

may continue to question the Council until the parties are satisfied. It often happens that a case is submitted to the Council several times.

The number of cases enquired into by the Council is about 2600 per annum (the population of the country is 5 million), of which approximately 30% concern intoxicated drivers (Table 1). Quite a number of these cases are complicated by the fact that, in addition to alcohol, the driver has also been under the influence of some psychotropic drug; neuroleptics, antidepressants and the minor tranquillizers all seem to potentiate directly the effect of alcohol, so that it is not a question of a summation effect only.

The number of psychiatric cases ranges between 800 and 1000 annually, corresponding to approximately 40% of the total. Owing to the complicated and time-consuming nature of these cases, they occupy a substantial part of the Council's time. The following categories predominate:

1. Cases involving mentally deviant criminals.
2. Before the Court decides whether a person who has been sentenced to detention in a mental hospital or in an institution for the feeble-minded can be discharged on parole, the Council will have to submit an advisory statement.
3. A patient retained in a mental hospital against his will can, according to Danish law, demand that his case be put before the Ministry of Justice or alternatively before the court. Prior to the court's decision all such cases are put before the Medico-Legal Council.
4. Finally the psychiatric section of the Council expresses its opinion in a series of cases pertaining to marriage and divorce of insane or mentally defective persons, and to alcoholic intoxication of drivers in whose case there may be a question of abnormal alcohol reaction, etc.

The annual reports of the Council, which can be supplemented by the reports of the Royal Health Board as far back as 1843, jointly provide a revealing picture of medico-legal evolution throughout a century and also give a convincing impression of the practical importance of the Medico-Legal Council. However, the picture would be incomplete if it were concealed that the Medico-Legal Council, in common with all such public institutions, has been exposed to criticism.

A drawback of the Medico-Legal Council has been said to be that it gives its opinions on the basis of the documents in the case without direct knowledge of the persons involved. It has been asserted that such an estimate may rest on a more uncertain foundation than the medical reports which form the basis of the opinions. If, however, the Council were in general to carry out direct examinations – which would be quite possible and which in fact happens in particular cases – the institution would assume impracticable dimensions. Nor is it correct that medical reports cannot be evaluated as they are, since the Council can in part check whether premises and conclusion agree and in part weigh up the desirability of the measures it is proposed to take. Finally, the Council is at liberty to request supplementary information or claim a new examination and statement if the material at hand is considered insufficient. It has also been claimed to be unsatisfactory that the opinions of the Council are issued in written form and are not followed up by spokesmen for the Council appearing in court in order to elaborate its views and answer pertinent questions. However, this criticism overlooks the fact that the Council is a college and that it would be contrary to its fundamental principles if single members or experts acted independently in the courts.

It has also been asserted that dissenting opinions are seldom recorded. It is said that scientists normally do not agree, and unanimous opinions must therefore often represent compromises between contrasting views, with which it might be of value for the courts as well as the parties to be acquainted. In the first place it may be said that while dissenting opinions occasionally, though seldom, occur, there are other ways of advancing the pros and cons underlying the opinions. It must also be maintained that it is necessary to attempt to get a consensus, as the choice between the possibilities at hand is otherwise referred to bodies essentially incompetent.

Thus there may be reasons to criticize certain aspects of the Danish Medico-Legal Council, but these should not overshadow the advantages of the system, which are in our opinion indisputable. First, the composition of the Council provides a far-reaching security that its statements rest on professional expert knowledge generally accepted by society. Consequently, the decisions of the court will as a rule be based on the advisory statements of the Council. This means that the court's use of expert witnesses, with the often dubious cross-examination of doctors whose impartiality may be questionable, is a practically unknown phenomenon in Denmark. Major emphasis should once more be placed upon the fact that the final advisory statement is thus given by experts who are in principle independent of the parties involved and of financial interests. Second, the existence of the Medico-Legal Council is in a great measure conducive to the establishment of uniform guidelines of forensic procedure in the different jurisdictions of the country. Not least, in relation to local psychiatric experts the Council has an important pedagogic function in the claims that it makes upon the quality of primary psychiatric examinations and certificates. Finally, it has been ascertained that over the years the Council has been able gradually to influence criminal-political evolution in Denmark seen from medical and psycho-iogical-psychiatric points of view. This must be regarded as the most valuable consequence of the Danish system, which has simultaneously resulted in harmonizing the relations between the legal and medical experts – relations which are in other countries governed by continuous conflict and tension.

A postscript on the discussions at the Cambridge Conference on Society, Psychiatry and the Law

MARTIN ROTH AND ROBERT BLUGLASS

The indivisibility of the problems of mental health

The indivisibility of the manifold aspects of mental health, 'the seamless web of the subject' in the words of Dr Margaret Somerville, was in evidence in all the discussion sessions during the Cambridge Conference on Society, Psychiatry and the Law.

The dismantling of many of the large mental hospitals and the total 'open door' policies pursued in most of those that remain in many parts of the world, the steadily growing number of mentally ill in the community, many of them homeless and isolated, the overcrowding of the prisons and the bottlenecks in the Special Hospitals such as Broadmoor, represent one facet of the problem. The radical critique of psychiatric hospitals and other institutions and their dehumanising effects, and the civil rights campaigns for the right to receive or to refuse psychiatric treatment and the right of offenders to opt for punishment without benefit of psychiatry, comprise another aspect. The tide of new legislation in relation to the care of the mentally ill in many countries and the mutual disenchantment that has evolved between psychiatry and the law within the last two decades make up a third part of the picture. All appear closely entangled with each other.

Reports from the United States, Canada and several European countries regarding the predicament of the growing number of mentally ill persons discharged in recent years from mental hospitals into the community depicted a situation consistent in its main features throughout the affluent parts of the world. A substantial proportion of those discharged have joined the ranks of the homeless and are to be found wandering the streets of the great cities, sleeping in railway stations and under bridges, filling the emergency and reception centres to overflowing. When accommodated in hostels or rooming-houses, the quality of medical care they receive is inadequate and ill-coordinated. Many are unemployed and there are few opportunities for occupation, diversion or recreation. The hostels and homes they occupy are usually located in the poorest quarters of the large cities and isolated from the community around. The institutionalisation, custodial care and dehumanisation of the large mental hospital have not ended; they have merely been transferred into the community.

Community care was and remains a liberal and progressive concept, but its scope and limitations have never been submitted to systematic enquiry. The lesson repeatedly taught in the history of the mental health services – that to build on lofty ideals, doctrines and untested theories alone, is to build on sand – had been forgotten. The reformers of the early part of the nineteenth century who created the first mental hospitals were inspired by the noble concepts of 'moral treatment'. They sought to rescue the pauper lunatics from the inhumanities of the workhouse, to transfer them to small institutions in which individualised patient care based on sound principles could be administered. Nor was John Conolly, one of the great pioneers of the movement, content merely to transfer patients from one institution to another. He laid the foundations of a domiciliary service with the aid of which he hoped to provide outpatient care for the majority of mentally ill people. He involved their relatives and friends in the treatment and initiated courses of training for attendants.

But the 'cures' announced in the early days of high enthusiasm proved devoid of foundation. There were no effective treatments for mental disorder at the time. Admissions swelled in numbers, the wards became oppressively overcrowded and the criteria for admission to mental hospital became increasingly stringent. But although by the end of the nineteenth century admission was limited to the most severe cases, the hospitals were compelled to accommodate an increasing tide of chronic pauper patients. The personal quality of the care and the family atmosphere that had prevailed in the small hospitals of the 1830s and 1840s gave place to a restrictive and coercive regime. The patients and the small staff of attendants were locked away from the world behind high walls, barred windows and a morbid culture borne of prejudice, fear and isolation.

The modern era in the United Kingdom began with the Mental Treatment Act of 1930 which allowed for voluntary admission and initiated the first outpatient services. The 15 to 20 years that followed the Second World War was a time of high optimism and progress. The high walls around the hospitals were torn down and the barred windows removed. The discovery of effective treatments for the most serious psychiatric illnesses together with programmes of activity, occupation and rehabilitation in mental hospitals, made possible the discharge of an increasing proportion of those admitted, as also a large number of chronic residents, into the community. Then in the early 1960s, by a sudden leap of the imagination without enquiry or calculation, the possibilities were seen as limitless. The total closure of large mental hospitals whose functions were to be taken over by the community services and by inpatient units in general hospitals, was incorporated as a principle of policy by the Department of Health. The dismantling of large hospitals began. Similar programmes of deinstitutionalisation were initiated in other countries, in some cases, as in the United States, on a vast scale.

But the community cared little or not at all. The wheel had turned full circle. By a strange irony many of those with chronic mental illness have returned to share the accommodation and fate of the rootless destitutes, the vagrants, the chronic alcoholics and the ageing recidivist offenders at the bottom of the social scale from whom they had been enabled to part company through the exertions of the early reformers of 150 years ago. The 'seamless web' of the subject was soon to become apparent. The effects of the increasing rates of discharge into the community have been felt throughout not only the mental health services but all spheres of social welfare. Professor Alan Dershowitz (quoted by Professor Stone) compared confinement to a balloon; squeezed in one place it sticks out in another. Lionel Penrose made the same point in 1939 when he noted the inverse correlation between the number of psychiatric beds and the number of prison places. Countries whose attitudes had grown more compassionate and enlightened had implemented new approaches towards aberrant behaviours previously regarded as wholly sinful and criminal and leaving no place for care or healing.

A considerable part of the discussion at the Conference was concerned with the effects of the steady increase in the prison population that has arisen through a number of parallel and related developments. Over the last 25 years there has been an escalation in the number of convictions of erstwhile occupants of mental hospitals. These convictions are often minor in nature but sometimes grave and requiring a measure of security during treatment. The number of available beds has in the meantime declined through closure, dismantling or contraction of the mental hospitals and the total 'open door' philosophy espoused by those that continue to admit new patients. In the UK the Special Hospitals alone (and in other countries their counterparts) have been prepared to admit and care for seriously disturbed or violent patients – whether or not charged with any offence – and in consequence they are all seriously overstretched. And as the contributions of Professor Gunn and Dr Hamilton among others make clear, a substantial proportion of the present prison population in the UK requires and is at times in urgent need of psychiatric care which cannot be provided in their present environment.

Dangerousness

It is in the United States that most of the enquiries on the prediction of dangerousness have been carried out and where its implications for decision-making in respect of compulsory admission to hospital and the disposal of offenders in courts of law have been most thoroughly explored. The participants from the United States and Canada were prominent in the discussions that developed around these and related themes.

A sharp dilemma is posed for those responsible for decisions in all areas regarding disposal of offenders in that the need to protect the community may clash with the obligation to respect the human rights of the offender to freedom and autonomy. For a psychiatrist expected to assume responsibility for the safety of patients and also answerable in some cases for any danger they may pose for the community, a 50% risk that an individual with a past record of violence will behave injuriously after release from hospital or prison may be judged unacceptably high. On the other hand from the point of view of a lawyer protecting the civil rights of a client estimated to have only one chance in two or three of avoiding dangerous conduct, depriving such a client of his freedom may appear to be doing him less than justice.

A few salient points from the discussions must suffice in this brief summary. A 40–50% risk of violent or dangerous behaviour within a year of release amounts to several thousand times the overall risk for individuals without a criminal record drawn from the population at large. Are communities prepared to tolerate or accept risks of this order, and if they are not is their attitude socially or morally defensible? A Civil Rights advocate would hold that in the light of the standards of civilisation and humanity to which they must aspire in the present day and age, communities must be prepared to accept such risks. The sense of outrage and vehement protest unleashed following a number of well-publicised acts of violence and murder by discharged patients and prisoners in large cities of the United States are accordingly condemned as unenlightened and intolerant.

A former judge of the Court of Appeal in the United Kingdom, Sir Patrick Browne, made the point that if there were to be a choice between a substantial risk of harm to members of a community on the one hand and on the other some hazard of injustice to an individual offender on the grounds that the risk he presented was statistical and therefore uncertain, a judge would have to come down on the side of the community rather than the individual. Judges in normal social circumstances cannot, he believed, adopt standards of justice in decision-making that are removed by more than a certain distance from the wishes, aspirations and modes of reasoning of ordinary people, or they will forfeit the community's confidence in, and respect for, the law.

Be this as it may, critics have questioned the justice and validity of preventive detention for those who have in the past committed dangerous offences, and have supported their case with the aid of a number of philosophical arguments. In the first instance the right of those to be protected from the risk of predatory and gratuitous attacks must be balanced against the right of individual offenders to protection from unjust and unnecessary deprivation of liberty. This principle would command wide assent. But the weight merited by individuals within the community who insist on their right to protection under the law and the human rights of potential offenders will vary from one case to the next, according to the relevant facts and circumstances.

According to Mrs Floud some authorities would regard preventive detention of offenders as an unjust violation of human rights and dignity even when it is virtually certain that they would inflict harm on others. Few participants were prepared to treat the claims of potential aggressors and potential victims in so uneven a manner.

Preventive measures could be further criticised, it is alleged, on the grounds that there is a substantial subjective element in the perception of dangerousness which by inflating the actual risk is liable to cause unjust invasion of the human rights of offenders. The subjective element in human fears is ever present and irreducible. It is not danger as assessed by some objective criterion but the manner in which it is perceived which generates fear and anxiety. In recent years a number of sexual murders of consistent pattern within an English county and, in another area, a succession of rapes which proved to be acts of revenge and humiliation and not just forceful intercourse, generated anxiety and panic that reached epidemic proportions among women in each community. The statistical risk to any individual may have been small. But the ability to estimate risk in precise and objective terms is rare, and in any case bears little relationship to the manner in which individuals, including those equipped with statistical knowledge, feel or behave when exposed to a source of danger they are helpless to control. Such widespread terror generated by a single murderer at large is disproportionate to the risk of collective or individual harm. But it cannot be discounted on that score. Communities have the right to be protected from anxiety and insecurity as well as actual physical attack.

The injustice of any preventive action taken in response to the collective claims of those whose particular rights and liberties are not directly threatened, that is on the basis of Professor Dworkin's concept of 'external preferences', is another philosophical argument invoked to question the justice of preventive measures against potential offenders on behalf of communities. However, it is not clear how the *directness* of the threat to individuals in a community who seek protection from danger can be objectively assessed.

Abstract philosophical systems of justice which have their starting point in a number of absolute and inalienable human rights have their part to play in the shaping of laws. But justice cannot be built upon a foundation of such principles alone. And the administration of the law has to be a far more pragmatic and flexible affair if it is to deserve the name of justice.

Actuarial prediction and clinical judgment of dangerousness

Mrs Floud drew a distinction between actuarial prediction of risk on the one hand and clinical judgment of it on the other. It was generally agreed that one should complement the other to make it possible to take account of the individual clinical features that are glossed over in any statistical computation of risk. Although the distinction is real it is doubtful whether the methods are conceptually entirely different in character. Clinical judgment is possible only on the basis of past experience of similiar individual cases in numbers sufficiently large to make generalisation of some kind possible. Judgments ostensibly made on the strength of the unique features of individuals are probably less intuitive and subjective than they appear. Faced with a person truly unique in respect of features relevant to dangerousness, the experienced psychiatrist can do no more than contemplate him in ineffable wonder and perplexity.

The subject is replete with paradoxes. Judges in the United States in particular have shown themselves increasingly influenced by the view that dangerousness is insufficiently predictable to be of value for decisions regarding the disposal of offenders. At the same time proof of dangerousness has been demanded to justify the compulsory commitment of patients to a psychiatric hospital.

The elevation of dangerousness to the status of a central criterion in the trial of offenders whose sanity or 'responsibility' is at issue has some strange consequences, exemplified in the outcome of the trial of John Hinckley, the would-be assassin of President Reagan. That Hinckley shot the President and had intended to kill him was not in doubt. However, the jury acquitted him on the grounds of insanity. After the trial Hinckley was to describe the psychiatric testimony that had been presented during the trial in the following terms: 'The defence doctors found me to be delusional, psychotic, schizophrenic and perhaps the most alienated young man they have ever examined. On the other hand, despite evidence to the contrary, the prosecution doctors said I merely had some personality problems and deserved to be punished with imprisonment.' As under the system of periodic review prevalent in the United States he would be eligible to be released after recovering from his insanity there was widespread public anxiety about the possibility of renewed danger to the President. As the Master of Balliol College, Oxford, has pointed out in his Blackstone Lecture (Kenny, 1983) this provoked the American magazine *Newsweek* to formulate a telling paradox. Once Hinckley was committed, it was open to his attorneys to argue that he should be released because he was no longer mentally ill. In support of this claim they could point to the testimony of the prosecution throughout the trial. The government lawyers, on the other hand, in order to ensure that he continued to be hospitalised, would have been able to appeal to the eloquent speeches of the defence lawyers to the effect that the accused was severely mentally ill.

Psychiatric testimony in the courts

The verdict of insanity in the case of Hinckley outraged the public in the United States. And the sharply contradictory diagnoses pronounced in courts of law by different experts in a succession of recent cases brought psychiatric testimony into disrepute. Indeed Mr Kenny is led to question whether the evidence in relation to which reputable witnesses are so often in conflict possesses the characteristics of *expert* evidence and whether psychiatry as depicted in courts of law 'displays the lineaments of a science'. He was doubtful also whether the psychiatric diagnosis, even when firmly established, is relevant to the actual issues in respect of which courts of law are expected to adjudicate.

Accounts of the manner in which psychiatric testimony is presented in courts of law in different countries represented at the Conference, favoured the view that much of the contradiction in the testimony provided by psychiatric witnesses is artificially generated by the adversarial system. In this connection the account by Professor Lunn of the role of the Danish Medico-Legal Council in cases that present a psychiatric aspect proved of particular interest. In its essentials the organisation and its methods of procedure are similar to those in operation in other Scandinavian countries. Responsibility for presenting evidence to the courts is assumed by three of the expert members of the Medico-Legal Council. Great pains are taken to ensure that all evidence relevant for the evaluation by the experts is placed before them, and the records are studied in detail. In most Scandinavian countries the opinion expressed is confined to a statement about the psychiatric diagnosis of the offender's disorder. The formulation is wider in scope in Denmark and includes a statement on 'responsibility' – for reasons that Professor Lunn has cogently explained in his paper. A diagnosis by the experts might for example take the form 'irresponsibility owing to psychosis'. On the strength of this opinion the courts would judge the offence in question as 'not punishable' and recommend detention in a mental hospital.

The main interest at the Conference centred on the almost invariable unanimity of the diagnoses presented to the courts by the Council, the rarity of the cases in which the disposal decided by the court was at variance with the implicit recommendation made, and the fact that the experts were virtually never brought into court for cross-examination. Although a number of reservations were expressed in the discussions regarding the acceptability of such procedures, the clarity and consistency of the testimony presented, and the authority that the Council commands in the courts and with the general public, presented a sharp contrast to the experiences of most Conference participants. Scandinavian practices and experience are clearly worthy of more detailed study by those working at the interface between the law and psychiatry.

Psychiatric explanations for aberrant behaviour and the law

Professor Villars Lunn emphasised that as the consequences of a diagnosis of 'psychosis' by a commission of the Medico-Legal Council were of fateful importance, it was made on the strength of very strict criteria. Psychotic disorders that arise after stresses of an extremely onerous nature or the acute illnesses of brief duration in individuals with personality disorder would not have qualified. It was plain that psychotic features of a highly specific kind had to be present to satisfy the criteria. They would have included such features as 'primary' delusions, experiences of passivity, perceptual disturbances and behaviour qualitatively distinct from normal patterns constituting a break in the continuity of the person's psychic life.

character are beyond the reach of empathy and psychological understanding in the sense of Jaspers and his predecessors in this tradition such as Dilthey.

In his searching analysis of the kinds of explanation advanced by psychiatrists to explain aberrant conduct Professor Walker found little use for the concept of 'understandability' in its implications for law breaking behaviour. He judged such formulations to have the character of 'possibility' explanations or 'probability' explanations although he was dubious about the latter in that they appeared to entail probabilities of a low or unspecifiable order. He cited the low prevalence of infanticide in the totality of women with puerperal depression as testifying to the weakness of the purported link between the emotional disorder and murder of an infant after childbirth.

It may be agreed that a puerperal psychotic depression in a woman who has committed infanticide does not constitute a sufficient cause or explanation for the murder. But her 'illness' has to be judged a necessary causal factor in that the great majority of women who commit infanticide suffer from a puerperal psychosis. Evidence for the specific link with such a depressive illness is provided by the effects of antidepressive treatment, which will usually bring the depression, and any compelling urges to hurt the child, under control within a short time.

The low prevalance of infanticide among women suffering from puerperal depression is of some relevance for the problem of its causation. But it is less telling as a piece of evidence, than comparison of the prevalance of infanticide in women suffering from a puerperal psychosis with that manifest in the same women during puerperal periods when they are mentally well, during the years that intervene between the births of their children and the segment of their life that follows the menopause. Infanticide at the age of, let us say, 30 years and within a few weeks of childbirth will commonly prove to be the only seriously violent or murderous form of conduct manifest in such a patient in the course of a long life.

It is surprising that in his attempt to discover 'crimes committed as a result of delusions which if true would have justified them in law. . . .' Nigel Walker did not come across an illustrative case of puerperal psychosis in view of the fact that some such patients may commit suicide or murder relatives as well as their new-born child.

Some of the disparity in the thinking of lawyers and criminologists on the one hand and psychiatrists on the other arises from the different manner in which we construe the term 'understanding' and the difficulty of defining this in precise terms. 'Understandability' cannot be assessed by objective means nor measured reliably. But this does not signify that it is nebulous or non-existent. Professor Walker stated that in an account of a man who had in a paranoid delusion killed his wife believing that she had been unfaithful to him, he could say to himself 'I see why he did it'. Psychiatrists would agree with him in some cases. But it is their inability to concede such an interpretation in others that leads them to make a diagnosis of paranoid schizophrenia rather than 'morbid jealousy' of a different character. A man of 39 detected a knowing expression on the face of a man who was a complete stranger but gazed at him for some seconds. He immediately interpreted the knowing look as convincing evidence that his wife was having a sexual relationship with this man and with a large number of others in the small town in which they lived, including incestuous intercourse with their 16 year old son. After he had murdered his spouse, he produced handkerchiefs and pieces of underwear in which he had detected large seminal stains. They were invisible to others and under forensic examination his suspicions proved to be groundless.

The 'understanding' that an observer may have in such a case is illusory. A 'primary' delusion as in the case summarised entails a leap in inference, and reasoning from a normal perception to an intense conviction that clashes with reality and resists all evidence to the contrary. Patients who recover from the psychosis in the course of which they have committed a murder while under the influence of a delusion will usually be bewildered, stricken and incapable of understanding what they had done. It should be added that the logic which holds that the 'insanity defense' should have validity only if the offence during a psychosis would have been justified in law if the underlying delusion had been true in fact, would be regarded by most psychiatrists as unacceptably rigid.

Some effects upon clinical and community practice

Professor Stone described the manifold adverse effects on the care of patients in community and hospital of the 'criminalisation' of psychiatric practice, the allocation to psychiatrists of a primary role in the control of violence and the protection of the public from it. This, he averred, was a 'policeman's role'.

In trying to estimate the risk that an individual might behave in an aggressive or violent manner, self-destructive behaviour has to be considered alongside violence towards others, for the two forms of conduct are to some extent correlated. Now the risk of consummated suicide in an individual case is as indeterminate as the chance of dangerous behaviour in an offender seeking an abridgement of his sentence. Yet there are a whole range of clinical features in the psychological profile of depressive and other patients that are generally accepted as providing forewarning of a high risk of suicide. Should a psychiatrist fail to anticipate self-destructive conduct in such cases he will be liable to be sued for negligence. Substantial damages have increasingly been awarded in recent years to the dependents and relatives. A similar situation obtains in respect of the risk of arson, violence or murder. The responsibility of a therapist for warning the potential victims of his patients has been embodied in the judgment relating to the Tarasoff case in the United States (1976). And psychiatrists have been penalised for alleged negligence in such cases in the UK among other countries. Yet the possibility of making valid or reliable predictions of dangerousness in clinical and forensic practice has been repeatedly called in question in recent years. Faced with such double-bind situations* there is a danger that those engaged in the practice of psychiatry will assume an increasingly defensive posture. There may be disinclination to take responsibility for the care or for the admission to hospital of those in whom examination reveals more than latent potentialities for violent or impulsive conduct.

Participants from the United States drew attention to a recent surge of withdrawal from the public sector of mental health practice. Despite the fact that violence does not in itself call for a psychiatric diagnosis an increasing number of uncontrollable persons who may also be untreatable in hospital under the constraints currently imposed by the law, have accumulated in psychiatric hospitals. In the meantime, many of those who would benefit from treatment but fail to qualify for compulsory commitment or for involuntary treatment by present-day criteria wander the streets without help or languish in hospital while their disease grows more chronic and refractory. The issues posed are of fateful importance for the welfare of those who suffer in mind and for the future of psychiatry and merit consideration in a widely representative international forum.

Competence to give informed consent

The right to refuse treatment was seen by Mr Gostin as an inalienable human right and its wide acceptance as such as an achievement of the human rights movement. There were disagreements

---

* Some instructive examples were given in Professor Helmchen's discussion of the laws governing the management of potentially suicidal patients in Germany. According to a provincial decision in Frankfurt-am-Main, confirmed by the Federal Supreme Court in 1977, in the case of such patients absolutely particular and concrete measures for their protection must be met. But involuntary treatment (except in an emergency, which is very narrowly defined) can be given only with the consent of a legal guardian who has to be appointed by a judge.

as to who should assume responsibility for taking decisions in matters of competence. Mr Gostin rejected the view that it should be the professional peers of psychiatrists. He favoured a lay body both for undertaking the review and for looking after patients' rights in general. American participants were inclined to leave responsibility to judges and courts of law while English and European non-psychiatric representatives favoured an independent consultant psychiatrist nominated by a Mental Health Commission as the kind of person best qualified to undertake the task.

The whole competency issue has significant implications for psychiatric medicine, where treatments have often to be administered to demented, delirious and partly conscious patients without prior consideration of their competence to give informed consent to refuse treatment. The discussion also has far-reaching implications for general medicine, for as Professor Bluglass pointed out neuroleptic, anxiolytic and sedative drugs are widely used in the management of severely ill patients in general hospitals. Who should undertake, he enquired, the assessment of competence in general medical cases? What would be the ethically correct procedure to adopt in a case of advanced mental deterioration? Should the decision be taken by a judge, a relative, a psychiatrist or a panel made up of lay representatives as well as professionals? The general feeling among British and Continental participants was that judges lacked the necessary knowledge to make assessments of mental competence. North American participants were on the whole inclined to favour the courts and judges in this role.

Imprisonment in place of hospital care
A prominent feature of recent decisions regarding the disposal of offenders has been the steep decline in the number of hospital orders and the parallel increase in the proportion of prison sentences in the case of individuals found guilty of manslaughter rather than murder on account of diminished responsibility owing to mental disorder. Mrs Suzanne Dell told the Conference of her recently completed investigation into all documents relating to diminished responsibility cases during the period 1966 to 1977 (253 cases after the exclusion of a small number). In 90% of cases doctors agreed about the question of diminished responsibility and disagreement in respect of diagnosis was confined to 8%. Despite the high levels of morbidity among those found guilty of manslaughter on grounds of diminished responsibility (one half were mentally ill at the time of the offence and a quarter were judged to have severe personality disorder), there was a progressive decrease over the period investigated in the

proportion of individuals in respect of whom hospital order recommendations were made. Serious overcrowding in Special Hospitals and the 'open door' policies of the local psychiatric hospitals were the main causes of these inappropriate placements. These findings make a powerful case for reform of the law and for early consideration by Parliament of the Butler Committee's report in the hope that its main recommendations are implemented at an early date.

Repeated reference was made during the Conference to the crisis that has been created by the overcrowding in Special Hospitals and the absence of alternative facilities such as were available in the past in local psychiatric hospitals for the management of persistently disturbed and dangerous patients whose care demands a certain measure of security. With the recent establishment of some more secure units some measure of relief is perhaps within sight. But the medical director of Broadmoor, Dr John Hamilton, appeared to share the doubts expressed by Parker and Tennent that regional secure units could solve the problem in the foreseeable future.

Psychiatric services within prisons

The creation of facilities for psychiatric treatment within the penal system was dear to the heart of the much-lamented late Dr Peter Scott. During the last 15 years of his life he held steadfastly to the view that the prisons were in dire need of a caring, therapeutic component to mitigate the harshness of an essentially punitive system. Such an innovation could have resolved some of the pressing problems discussed in the previous section. As Professor Gunn indicated, however, his conception was at variance with recommendations of the late Professor Trevor Gibbens and his colleagues. They believed that the most hopeful approach towards the integration of mentally abnormal offenders into the community would be to treat them as ordinary psychiatric patients within general psychiatric hospitals. According to this view, most offenders should be dealt with by general psychiatrists or generalists with a special interest in forensic work. A further complication foreseen by Professor Gunn is that the establishment of social and psychiatric services within the prison system might actually encourage the courts and society to divert more mentally abnormal people there. Prison would be the wrong kind of environment for them. A caring and compassionate atmosphere and the objectives of healing and rehabilitation are indispensable components in any psychiatric service worthy of the name. And it would be difficult or impossible to introduce such features in the forseeable future into prisons as they are at present.

Concluding remarks

The debate will continue for an indefinite time ahead. For in its essentials the issues addressed in Cambridge have not changed since they were first presented at the dawn of civilisation. We deal with painful and obdurate dilemmas and contradictions which brook no simple solution. Society's ambiguously poised attitudes towards the mentally ill were already evident at the beginning of recorded history when the same combination of care and compassion for the insane, on the one hand, and demonology with its persecutions and tortures, were already in evidence. As far as acts of antisocial violence are concerned the ambivalence was different in character. This is well exemplified by rape, which has been execrated and punished in all cultures in times of peace. But war transforms the face of justice and mortality. As Szent-Gyorgi (1963) has pointed out the rape of the Sabine women was depicted as one of the glorious victories of ancient Rome.

REFERENCES

Kenny, A. (1983). The expert in Court. (Revised version of the Seventh Blackstone Lecture.) *Law Quarterly Review*, 99, 197–216.
Tarasoff v. *Regents of the University of California*, 551 P.Zd 334 (1976).